Praise for *12 Weeks to Self-Healing*

"12 Weeks to Self-Healing: Transforming Pain through Energy Medicine by Candess Campbell, PhD is one of the best books I've encountered. It explores the mysteries of the healing process in a beautiful, yet easy, way to understand. The book offers tools and techniques that will help most people with chronic pain conditions. I have to compliment the author in her ability to combine well known medical/physical concepts and principles with the less known, more mysterious, abstract metaphysical/spiritual concepts. I have no hesitation in recommending this book to almost anybody, but in particular to those people with chronic illnesses. As a medical doctor, I have to say that the medical facts are well researched and I definitely endorse this book as another therapeutic tool and would not hesitate to recommend it to many of my own patients."

— **David Sandoval M.D.**, rheumatologist

"I love your book! I am so happy to be back in it ... amazing learning potential and such a wonderful shift in style. It reminds me of peaches. I know that I like them, but I always forget how MUCH I like them until I sink my teeth right back into one. Juicy, sweet, simple, and healthy. Just like 12 Weeks!"

— **Pamela Maliniak**, editor and intuitive writing coach of *12 Weeks to Self-Healing: Transforming Pain through Energy Medicine* and other works, such as *The Bliss Mistress Guide to Transforming the Ordinary Into the Extraordinary* and *Breaking Free from Critical Addiction*

"If you're tired of feeling sick and powerless, grab a copy of **12 Weeks to Self-Healing: Transforming Pain through Energy Medicine** by Candess Campbell, Ph.D. This book offers a comprehensive explanation of the mind-body connection and presents practical ways to break old habits that lead to illness. As an energy worker, Campbell understands the dimensions beyond accepted Western thinking, and yet is well-versed in the advances of modern medicine. This is a book that will help people transform their lives."

— **Dana Taylor**, author of *Ever-Flowing Streams*
SupernalLiving.com

"Healing is not just a physical journey; it is also a mental, emotional, and spiritual journey. In **12 Weeks to Self-Healing: Transforming Pain through Energy Medicine**, Candess Campbell has gathered a thorough compendium of resources and exercises to help you tap into your own power to heal or transform your relationship to pain. Following her 12-week outline, you are sure to find tools to assist you on your journey."

— **Carol Woodliff**, shaman & intuitive coach, and author of *From Scared to Sacred: Lessons in Learning to Dance with Life*

"Candess Campbell has a gem of a book that will touch your mind, heart, and soul. Anyone experiencing pain will be nourished by her wisdom, and touched by her compassion. Her unique combined experience in psychology and energy work has given her distinct knowledge that really changes live. This is integrative medicine at it's finest, and provides huge insights!"

— **Jill Weadick**, spiritual teacher

"*Proven methods distilled from the author's life experience will jump start your personalized program of self-healing. Even as a seasoned Energy Healer for over 35 years, I discovered new areas of practical information. Candess lifelong passion to bridge allopathic and energy/vibrational medicine crystalizes in* **12 Weeks to Self-Healing.***"*

— **Michael David Lawrience**, author of *The Secret for Freedom from Drama, Trauma, and Pain*

"*I have been astonished by the quality of content Candess has provided related to her book* **12 Weeks to Self Healing***. As someone who lived severely disabled by CFS/ME for over 14 years, I am selective about who I listen to on the subject of healing. I want someone to acknowledge the difficulties of illness and move us forward from where we are. I want practical exercises that I can apply to my life. Candess does all this and more.*"

— **Katherine T Owen**, author of *It's OK to Believe*
www.a-spiritual-journey-of-healing.com

"*From the very beginning, Dr. Candess Campbell balances clinical information with practical suggestions for emotional and physical pain relief. She explains, in real-life terms, how our daily choices can impact our physical health. Most importantly, she shares ideas for holistic and integrative solutions that can work without negative side effects, starting today!*"

— **Camille Leon**, founder and executive director,
The Holistic Chamber of Commerce
www.HolisticChamberOfCommerce.com

12 Weeks to Self-Healing:

Transforming Pain through Energy Medicine

Vesta Enterprises Press
Spokane, Washington 99201

This publication contains the opinions and ideas of the author. It is intended to provide helpful and informative material. It is sold with the understanding that the information in the book is generic and does not replace any formal medical or psychiatric treatment. The author and publisher are not engaged in rendering personal medical, mental health, health, or any other kind of professional services. The reader should consult his or her medical, mental health, or health provider before adopting any of the suggestions in this book or drawing inferences from it.

The author and publisher specifically disclaim all responsibility for any liability, loss or risk, personal or otherwise, that is incurred as a consequence, directly or indirectly, of the use and application of any of the contents within this book.

12 Weeks to Self-Healing:

Transforming Pain through Energy Medicine

Candess M. Campbell, PhD

Edited by: Pamela Maliniak

This book is dedicated to my mom, Shirley Jennie Topper.

Had I known then what I know now …

Foreword

12 Weeks to Self-Healing is unlike other books in its genre. As I read the manuscript, I was impressed by how well the book is written, how effectively the book reveals the hidden causes that undergird the pain and sorrow felt by so many, and how gently (yet efficiently) the healing process is promoted.

Most self-help books these days are simply easy turn-and-learn pages that say nothing real but deliver many glittering generalities. The fact is, there is a real miasma in the self-help industry today that revolves around the idea of "tell them what they want to hear." As such, there is an abundance of popular quotations and well-recited advice that simply sounds good but fails to empower. It may make one feel good for a while, it may inspire for a moment, it may even elevate a mood for a day or so—but these glowing, emotionally appealing words do no more than make self-help junkies out of their fans.

Dr. Candess Campbell's *12 Weeks to Self-Healing* raises the bar for self-help books. As you turn the pages, you will discover the full power of the tools and techniques she provides. No matter the life circumstances that have brought you to this book, you will benefit from the read, even if it is just to better understand those in pain—emotional and/or physical pain. Indeed, this is a book for everyone, for we have all known pain of one sort or another, and we all know others who are in pain.

12 Weeks to Self-Healing is an apt title for a book that promises and delivers exactly what the title suggests. I encourage you to immerse yourself in a journey that will yield great personal rewards!

Eldon Taylor, PhD, FAPA
New York Times Bestselling Author
Talk Radio Host

Table of Contents

List of Figures

Acknowledgements

Giving birth to *12 Weeks to Self-Healing: Transforming Pain through Energy Medicine* was an intense and exhilarating process! My heartfelt gratitude goes to my editor, Pamela Maliniak, not only for her unwavering playful, validating, and gentle support, but also for her setting necessary deadlines that kept me on my toes. Her supportive emails were invaluable. Pam's incredible ability not only to edit, but also to connect one stream of thought to another and to nudge me to deepen in some areas and to be concise in others, took this manuscript to a higher level.

Without my virtual assistant Caroline Hansen, who assisted me from the time this book was a dissertation, I would not have been able to complete either one. She supported me in everything from organizing to formatting and marketing. Her expert ability, her readiness to stay with the process and persevere to the end, as well as her assistance in keeping my business growing during the process was incredible.

Thanks to Pamela J. Hunter for the magnificent book cover, to Joanne Wilkinson for the graphic idea and her support in my Mastermind Group, and to the other creative and beautiful women of my Mastermind Group. This includes Susie Leonard Weller, Valerie Lipstein, Doreen Desmond, Joanne Wilkinson and Victoria Love; they have been supportive and uplifting. Over the years, many generous readers have helped me, and I am eternally grateful to you all!

Genuine gratitude goes to Alex Docker, for his continual guidance, feedback, and gentle support through the coursework that led to my expertise as a hypnotherapist. Brian Walsh, my dissertation advisor, gave me superb supervision and patience throughout the writing process. His incredible attention to detail shifted how I saw myself and helped me to understand the value of quality.

More recently, I have had the honor of becoming acquainted with Eldon Taylor. I am grateful to him, not only for meeting with me and sharing his experience as a writer and writing my foreword, but also for being a Hay House author who has continually awakened us with over 25 years of researching the power of the mind and developing scientifically proven methods to use in order to enhance the quality of our lives. His presence in my life has given me hope and aspiration!

Blessings to my clients over the last thirty years who have inspired me to learn, grow, and serve. I have been so blessed to work with adolescents in halfway homes and transitioning from juvenile detention; adolescents and adults struggling to gain recovery from alcohol and drugs in treatment programs; Native American adolescents who suffered from addiction as well as family conditions that prevented them from having a fair chance; men and women in the Federal Correctional System who were arrested and taken from their families for minor drug charges and placed in a federal camp for five years during the War on Drugs; men and women whose lives were disrupted due to trauma from childhood and as adults; and my many clients who came to me for spiritual readings and spiritual direction. I appreciate you all!

Without my dear friend Cheyenne Mendel, I would not have been able to balance my own life, and I love and cherish her for being my friend more than she knows. Thanks to Cheyenne and Carol Hilgers for their support in our weekly group that gently and lovingly lifted and guided me. Support from my treasured friend Dr. Gilbert Milner has been miraculous and sustained me through my health crisis and inner process. I am especially grateful to him for taking me through a hypnotic process to remember the details from the trauma I suffered at age fourteen that resulted in a near death experience (NDE) and for his patience as I sat with him week after week, resistant to meditation, until he guided me to Sri Ramana Maharshi, who has been a miracle in my life since.

Playful thanks go to my family who made fun of me for my beliefs most of my life. They motivated me to find a larger audience, and I love them dearly for not taking me seriously.

Finally, devoted and humbled thanks to E. C.

Preface

I was inspired to write this book after having worked with a client of mine. A woman in her fifties came to me directly from the psychiatric ward of a local hospital; she had been admitted because of severe depression and a threat to hurt herself. This woman suffered from rheumatoid arthritis and had been a victim of childhood sexual abuse. Initially, I had her read *The Artist's Way*, by Julia Cameron, to help in her process.[1] Many of the tools in Cameron's book were tools I had used for years, and this motivated me to write my own book on healing emotional and physical pain. Through the counseling process and these tools, my client began her journey back to her healthy Self.

Part One

Evaluate Your Situation

"The power of belief, the absolutely awesome incredible power of belief, is the genie in your life. Let me say that again: the absolutely awesome incredible power of belief, is the genie in your life."

– Eldon Taylor

How to Use This Book

In this book, you will find tools and exercises that will be helpful in your healing process. Make no mistake, self-healing is a step-by-step process, in which each small change builds to affect a considerable life difference.

To that end, I would like to introduce the amygdala. In a coaching class I took called Body-Mind Coaching Tools for Wellness, Dr. Lauree Moss shared from the book *One Small Step Can Change Your Life: The Kaizen Way* about the amygdala, a part of our brain that controls the fight-or-flight response.[1,2] She detailed the importance of not "waking up" the amygdala while making changes in your life (such as this self-healing), in order to avoid putting yourself in fight-or-flight while doing so.

From my own experience, and that which I've witnessed in clients, the fight response can appear to be an anger response or a response of resistance. The flight response, on the other hand, can include hiding, avoiding, or even feeling paralyzed. In the process of reading *12 Weeks to Self-Healing: Transforming Pain through Energy Medicine,* as you integrate and assimilate information and use the tools to begin new behaviors, I encourage you to be gentle with yourself—and, as much as you can, don't wake up the amygdala.

There is a membership website associated with this book, **http://www.12WeekstoSelfHealing.com**, where you can find audios and lesson plans connected with each week, as well as interviews with guest speakers on the subjects I discuss within this book. The online membership website also provides you with a personal journal. There are additional online resources available, as outlined in the appendix. Feel free to join with others in the healing process by joining the Facebook Group called 12 Weeks to Self-

Healing at **http://on.fb.me/Candess.** There are also resources on my website at **http://www.CandessCampbell.com**.

You will notice that I reference the website often, offering many resources. While you would be greatly helped by these resources, do not feel concern if you don't use the Internet, because this book gives you all the tools you need. If this is the case and you do decide to start using the Internet in conjunction with your self-healing, you may consider asking a friend or support/daily person, child, or grandchild to access my site for you. This might be fun! Also, most libraries are equipped with computers and Internet and some with classes as well.

The journal process below is separate from the online journal process. I encourage you to begin the one below now, using it as you read this book. It will carry through to your everyday life.

Journal Process

One of my favorite healing tools is journaling and free writing. I have journaled for over thirty years and find it to be not only helpful but also fun. Several years ago, I gained major insight through journaling while working with clients in my office. I began experiencing pain in my neck and shoulders and continually changed positions to get more comfortable, but nothing helped. After a few days of this pattern, the pain became worse. I realized there must be something within myself I was not addressing.

The next day, after seeing clients, I picked up my journal, set the timer for twenty minutes, and began writing. Surprisingly, I found that my whole journal entry was about a situation with one of my daughters. Once I had exhausted the twenty minutes, I felt more relaxed and as if I had accomplished something positive. I checked in with my body and found the pain was gone. Even though I have used this process many times, I am always amazed at how simple it is to heal pain through becoming aware and using tools such as journaling and free writing.

To start, choose a notebook. I suggest one that is not expensive, one in which you can be messy and just write. I usually give clients a spiral notebook from my supply that I purchase in fall back-to-school sales. You can also use a three-ring binder with loose paper.

Second, find a pen that writes fast or that you particularly enjoy using. It's difficult to write for twenty minutes or longer with a pen that drags, sputters, or loses ink flow. Keep two or three pens easily accessible so you don't run out of ink.

You may also decide to use your computer to journal. I suggest you try both handwriting and computer journaling before you make the final decision. You may even decide to use both. Once you are ready, follow the steps below:

1. Set a timer for twenty minutes or commit to four full pages of notebook-sized paper.

2. Start with a sentence stem, like the following:

    If I were a bird …
    What frustrates me the most is …
    What I really want in my life is …

3. Continue writing for twenty minutes. Don't worry about punctuation or spelling—just keep your pen moving. If you are stuck, simply write

the words "I am stuck" or "I don't know what to write" repeatedly, until something else comes up.

If you find it difficult to write this way, I mentioned above that you can also free write on your computer. To do so, use the same process, including the sentence stems, commitment of time or pages, and typing without worry regarding grammar or spelling. When free writing, writing with a pen and paper is my first choice because I can access parts of myself I do not access on the computer, but the choice is yours.

According to Natalie Goldberg, author of *Writing Down the Bones*, you will probably start writing about something that is on the surface, such as what you are doing at the moment or have to do today.[3] You may move then into resistance ("I don't want to do this," "My hand hurts," "This is boring," etc.), and eventually you transition into what is really going on deep within you. It may take three or four sessions to get to the point where you access this deeper information, but don't give up. This is a commitment to healing and connecting with your Self!

Several years ago, the morning news reported on a study by Smyth, Stone, Hurewitz, and Kaell, published in the *Journal of the American Medical Association* (JAMA), showing study participants were able to reduce their symptoms of asthma and rheumatoid arthritis through writing. This study concluded:

> Patients with mild to moderately severe asthma or rheumatoid arthritis who wrote about stressful life experiences had clinically relevant changes in health status at 4 months compared with those in the control group. These gains were beyond those attributable to the standard medical care that all

participants were receiving. It remains unknown whether these health improvements will persist beyond 4 months or whether this exercise will prove effective with other diseases.[4]

I was delighted to read this, having known the healing properties of journaling in my own life experience for years!

Week One: Evaluate Your Situation

Everyone's experience is different. Now that you are ready to connect more deeply with yourself, the first thing to do is to evaluate your situation. When you don't feel well, it's easy to be overwhelmed and have a difficult time figuring out what is happening. The tools I provide this week will help you evaluate where you are and where to begin.

As previously mentioned, I provide resources and suggestions in this book; however, I understand that none of this is helpful without corresponding behavior. In my own life, I have found that reading the suggestions of other people has proven quite motivating. Using this book as a workbook will help you continue on your journey of self-healing. It will also help you assess your progress.

The first goal is getting from the beginning of this book to the end — this may be well assisted in having support. You can use the online membership website and/or the Facebook page I've already mentioned to connect with others and share support. You can also use this book with a friend, a life coach, or a mental health counselor.

When you make the commitment to yourself to complete this process and find support, you will be amazed by the rate of your progress. If you have not joined in any online groups before and decide to do so here, you may be surprised at the incredible support you will find with others in this online environment. I have several groups in which I participate, share, and gain support. My new online friends are not only beneficial but they have also become dear to me.

Cognitive Behavioral Theory

Cognitive behavioral therapy focuses on the importance of your thinking in relationship to your feelings. Although there are several cognitive behavioral theories, in this book I will focus on William Glasser's *Choice Theory*.[1] I became certified in choice theory in 1997 through the William Glasser Institute. D. Barnes Boffey developed a model from Glasser's work and published it in his book, *Reinventing Yourself*.[2]

Let's begin by understanding how Boffey's model describes each human existing as a "total behavior system." He shows the ways in which you behave through your doing, thinking, feeling, and physiology. Once you understand and practice this, you will eventually no longer need to write it down on the map found below. Instead, you will begin to complete the process in your mind. As an example, let's imagine a disturbing situation.

The situation I describe below is for demonstration purposes for you to understand the model of the Total Behavior Map. In your own personal life, other choices may be more appropriate, which I will discuss in Week Seven.

Alice suffers from chronic joint pain. She just turned fifty years old. Her daughter, Amy, lives several hundred miles away and forgot Alice's birthday. Amy generally calls weekly, but Alice didn't get a call this week. Alice has just finished reading a novel in which the daughter stopped talking to her mother because of unresolved feelings from childhood, and Alice starts to wonder why her own daughter didn't call. In addition, Alice recently missed an appointment with the doctor because the neighbor who takes her failed to show. Moreover, Alice didn't tell her friends about her birthday for fear of bothering them. She figured they were busy with their own lives, and she has been in so much pain lately that she doesn't really have the energy to do anything celebratory anyway. Now, having spent her birthday alone, Alice finds that the pain in her joints has increased, and she feels angry and hurt.

Look at Figure 1, the Total Behavior Map.

TOTAL BEHAVIOR MAP

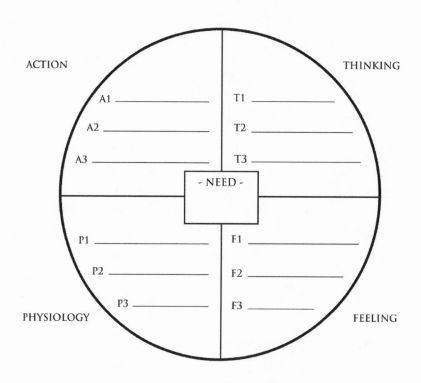

NAME THIS TOTAL BEHAVIOR

Figure 1 Total Behavior Map

Note: from *Reinventing Yourself*, 3rd printing 1997
D. Barnes Boffey, Ed.D.
Available from New View Publications, Chapel Hill, NC
info@newviewpublications.com. 1-800-441-3604.[3]

The top left of the circle is labeled *Action*. The top right is *Thinking*, the bottom left is *Physiology*, and the bottom right is *Feeling*.

Let's take a closer look at this situation. What might Alice be *doing*? Maybe she's not rescheduling her appointment with the doctor and not answering her phone or making any calls. She may be isolating. What is she *thinking*? She may be thinking that she doesn't care anyway. She would rather be alone because it's too much work to get together with people, and they don't understand what it feels like to be in pain. In her mind, Alice may label her daughter as being selfish. She focuses on the thought that she has spent her whole life caring for others, and now she's alone and no one seems to care.

What might Alice be *feeling* when doing these behaviors and thinking these thoughts? My best guess would be that she's feeling angry, hurt, sad, and maybe even a little vengeful. This vengeful feeling is probably turned inward, and Alice may be choosing not to eat, to eat more than she wants, or even to eat food she doesn't want. The more she feels these feelings, the more her joints ache (*physiology*), the more she isolates, and the more she engages in repetitive negative thoughts (*thinking*), which together manifest as ill health. It becomes a cycle of pain.

Glasser's cognitive theory explains that all behaviors are directed toward getting basic needs met. Other than survival, we have the need for the following: (1) love and belonging, (2) power and worth, (3) freedom, and (4) fun. Which needs do you suppose Alice is trying to meet with her behavior?

It appears that she wants a sense of love and belonging from her daughter. What she wants from her neighbor could also be considered love and belonging, but I imagine it includes some freedom as well. After all, wouldn't it be liberating for Alice to get out into the world and to her appointment? The need here could also be related to survival. Alice may be frightened about her health and feel it necessary to have her doctor check on a particular symptom. In addition, if her friends had been aware of her birthday, perhaps the need for fun would've been fulfilled.

Alice, like many of us, is stuck in a pattern of behavior. We attempt to get our needs met, but we fail to make choices that will allow us to actually reach those needs. Because *we are so unconscious of our own individual processes*, we begin to believe we have no choice and no control. We abandon our ability to manifest change; we live out of habit.

Let us look at how Alice could have chosen to otherwise handle this situation in a way that might've better met her needs. When Alice's birthday came and went without being recognized by a call from Amy or attention from her friends, Alice could have behaved differently. What if she had picked up the phone and called her daughter? She might have learned that Amy and the grandchildren were sick and that her daughter had been up all night caring for the family, causing her to sleep through the day. She might have found that, because she was so ill, Amy could barely talk and was anxiously waiting until the next day to call. Alice may have responded with understanding instead of feeling hurt and angry.

Had Alice made this call and understood how difficult the prior night had been for her daughter, what might her thoughts have been like? Perhaps she would think about how lucky she is to have missed the flu this year. She knows she has some pain, but she also knows it's manageable. Feeling grateful, she may have called her dear friend. In the course of the call, she might have told the friend about her daughter's situation and casually mentioned that it was her birthday. With this compassionate doing, thinking, and feeling behavior that results in calling her daughter and her friend, Alice's perception of the whole situation is altered. She might think that this is a good day. She might still miss her daughter and grandchildren, but the sadness would likely not affect her joints the way anger did. Additionally, in understanding her daughter's circumstances, perhaps the absence of anger would leave Alice's mind free to consider the possibility of celebrating her birthday in another way—or even on another day. This, in turn, offers the excitement of something fun to which she can look forward.

Let's turn our attention to the neighbor who was supposed to take Alice to the doctor. Being aware of how satisfying it had been to call her daughter, Alice might have decided (*behavior*) to call her neighbor as well. The neighbor might have apologized profusely. She might have explained that she had placed the appointment in her online calendar and that the computer had crashed. Perhaps she would have made it clear that she was truly sorry to have disappointed Alice—and then remembered it was also Alice's birthday. It's possible that she would have told Alice she would love to take her to dinner and a movie to celebrate. The two women could have rescheduled the medical appointment, had a lovely dinner, and watched an upbeat movie. Alice could have ended up having a great day after all.

Can you see the difference between the two scenarios based upon the choices Alice made in doing, thinking, and feeling, which also affect physiology? It's not difficult to see the results of the decisions in Alice's life. Now it is time to look at your own responses and how you can make better choices.

The situation I have described is simply one to assist you in understanding how to change the patterns that no longer work in your life today. These responses are usually developed from past events. There are definitely times in your life that reframing the situation is not the first action you will take. There are also times when the ones we love do not respond in healthy and rational ways. It may then be more effective to set boundaries and create relationships that are more satisfying, ones in which you can get your needs met. When that is the case, it is important to learn to detach and be sure to care for yourself. I address setting boundaries and self-care later in this book.

If you find yourself having a difficult time being positive and changing your thinking, allow yourself to be where you are and move from there. These patterns have taken a long time to develop and will change over time. Just love yourself where you are. Be gentle with yourself and know we all have room for growth, we are all in process, and small steps make a big difference.

Make some copies of the Total Behavior Map and practice. It helps to start with a less intense situation or disturbance, one that does not have a big charge. What I mean by *charge* is the level of reactivity with which you respond to the situation. Do you think about it several times a day or just occasionally? When you think about it, do you feel a knot in your stomach and lump in your throat, or does it just feel slightly frustrating? Do you immediately feel sad, or does your pain increase as you think about it? Later, after you've had some practice, you can work with more daunting disturbances.

The way in which you deal with your behaviors—your doing, thinking, and feeling—can affect your emotional state as well. This week, I am offering you some tools to assess whether you suffer from depression and/or anxiety related to your pain. It is difficult to tell sometimes whether the depression and/or anxiety caused the pain or vice verse. In his 2008 book, *Magnificent Mind at Any Age*, Daniel G. Amen clarifies, "One common misconception is that anxiety and depression are separate problems. They actually run together 70 percent of the time."[4] If you find you have some of the symptoms listed, it is imperative that you contact your physician, as these symptoms can be related to a medical illness. In fact, Amen further notes, "Thyroid abnormalities, anemia, sleep apnea, brain injuries, and certain medications can all cause these problems."

Take some time to go through the evaluations below, and I will then provide you with some solutions to assist with the treatment of depression and anxiety.

Depression

There are many symptoms of depression, and the intensity and duration of the symptoms determine the severity of the problem. Depression ranges from mild to severe. Please take the following simple test to see if you suffer from depression symptoms:

Mark the one answer that most closely matches how you have been feeling for the last two weeks or more.

- I feel sad or unhappy …

    A. Never
    B. Rarely
    C. Sometimes
    D. Very often

E.   Most of the time

- I feel tired, I don't have much energy, and/or I don't do as much as I used to do …

  A.   Never
  B.   Rarely
  C.   Sometimes
  D.   Very often
  E.   Most of the time

- I am discouraged about my life and my future …

  A.   Never
  B.   Rarely
  C.   Sometimes
  D.   Very often
  E.   Most of the time

- I cry or feel like crying …

  A.   Never
  B.   Rarely
  C.   Sometimes
  D.   Very often
  E.   Most of the time

- I feel uneasy, restless, or irritable …

  A.   Never
  B.   Rarely
  C.   Sometimes
  D.   Very often
  E.   Most of the time

- I have trouble sleeping (either sleep more than usual, sleep less than usual, feel unable to fall asleep, fall asleep and wake up one or two hours early and cannot get back to sleep) …

  A. Never
  B. Rarely
  C. Sometimes
  D. Very often
  E. Most of the time

- My appetite is greater or less than usual …

  A. Never
  B. Rarely
  C. Sometimes
  D. Very often
  E. Most of the time

- I am not as interested in other people or activities as I used to be …

  A. Never
  B. Rarely
  C. Sometimes
  D. Very often
  E. Most of the time

- I do not feel pleasure in things I used to enjoy …

  A. Never
  B. Rarely
  C. Sometimes
  D. Very often
  E. Most of the time

- I have lost interest in sex …

  A. Never
  B. Rarely
  C. Sometimes
  D. Very often
  E. Most of the time

- I have difficulty making decisions …

  A. Never
  B. Rarely
  C. Sometimes
  D. Very often
  E. Most of the time

- I can no longer concentrate …

  A. Never
  B. Rarely
  C. Sometimes
  D. Very often
  E. Most of the time

- I feel inadequate, like a failure or worthless …

  A. Never
  B. Rarely
  C. Sometimes
  D. Very often
  E. Most of the time

- I feel guilty without a rational reason and blame or criticize myself …

A. Never
B. Rarely
C. Sometimes
D. Very often
E. Most of the time

- I have lost confidence in myself and feel that things always go wrong or will go wrong no matter what I do …

  A. Never
  B. Rarely
  C. Sometimes
  D. Very often
  E. Most of the time

- I feel like I am being punished or expect to be punished …

  A. Never
  B. Rarely
  C. Sometimes
  D. Very often
  E. Most of the time

- I have suicidal thoughts …

  A. Never
  B. Rarely
  C. Sometimes
  D. Very often
  E. Most of the time

(If you have suicidal thoughts, even if you don't have a plan, it's imperative that you contact a local medical doctor or mental health professional.)

If you checked *Very often, Most of the time,* or *Sometimes* in several of these questions, you are at risk for depression and may have dysthymic disorder. Dysthymia is a low-grade depression lasting for at least two years, during which time you experience symptoms similar to those of depression, but you do not have what would be diagnosed as major depression. There are other disorders you may screen for as well, including bi-polar disorder. Bi-polar disorder has depressive symptoms as well as manic symptoms, which are periods of excessive happiness, excitement, irritability, restlessness, increased energy, and decreased need for sleep.

Diagnoses like these are based on a group of symptoms. The good news is that help is available. Assessing the problem is the beginning of healing. After completing this evaluation process, please contact your medical doctor or a local mental health counselor to assess more clearly the extent of your depression. You may want to take this book to your counselor or doctor and have him or her help you to work through it. Depression causes a lack of motivation, and your counselor or doctor can help you stay focused and on track in this healing process.

Although all healing is self-healing, part of this self-healing is reaching out for appropriate help. Women and men who are depressed or in chronic pain often ask for help from those who either do not know how to help or cannot help. The depressed person then feels powerless and stops asking for help. A mental health counselor, a doctor, or a support group are all appropriate resources to ask for help, but the best choice for your support system may not become clear until you have worked with the person for a short time.

Working with clients over time, I have noticed that those who suffer from depression are often focused on the past. Learning to stay in present time has been helpful. You can expect to find tools in this book to help you learn and pattern living in the present moment.

Disclaimer: This preliminary screening test for depressive symptoms does not replace, in any manner, a formal psychiatric evaluation. It is designed to give a preliminary idea about the presence of depressive symptoms.

Anxiety

Again, the purpose of this self-evaluation is to help you organize your symptoms so you can better understand your experience and communicate clearly with your health care providers, such as your physician, acupuncturist, massage therapist, and mental health counselor.

Anxiety is another disorder that may exist in conjunction with chronic pain. As is true of depression, anxiety can range from mild to severe. Anxiety disorder is characterized by excessive, exaggerated anxiety. People worry about everyday life events and continually fret about their family, work or school, money, or health. They tend to expect that something bad will happen. When the anxiety is severe, it interferes with their daily life, activities, and relationships.

Check the symptoms below that you experience on a regular basis:

I worry more often than not.

I experience excessive tension.

Others say I have an unrealistic view of problems.

I feel restless or edgy.

I experience irritability.

I have excessive muscle tension.

I have frequent headaches.

I perspire more than others for no apparent reason.

I have difficulty concentrating.

I feel nauseous.

I go to the bathroom frequently.

I feel tired or fatigued.

Several factors can contribute to anxiety, including genetics, brain chemistry, and environmental stresses. Some believe the weight on genetics as they relate to anxiety levels is a myth and that our learned beliefs have a greater influence than our genetics. In the brain, the levels of neurotransmitters (chemical messengers) that communicate from one cell to another may affect anxiety. Environmental factors—stress from events like job loss or change, relationship issues, financial issues, or loss of a loved one— can also create anxiety. Previously, I stated that clients who are depressed often focus on the past. Clients who struggle with anxiety are often focused on the future. Learning to stay in present time has been helpful for both groups.

Check the statements below that apply to you:

I tend to worry more days than not and have difficulty controlling the worry.

I feel restless or on edge.

I am easily fatigued.

I have a difficult time concentrating.

My mind goes blank often.

I tend to be irritable, or others say I am irritable.

My muscles are tense.

I have difficulty falling asleep, staying asleep, or I have restless sleep.

When assessing possible symptoms of anxiety, it's also important to assess your consumption of caffeine. Coffee, tea, soft drinks, and chocolate all contain caffeine and may create these symptoms. If you need to stop using caffeine for a time to determine whether it is contributing to your symptoms, you may want to change to a high quality green tea. Green tea has enough caffeine that you will probably avoid withdrawal while still being able to assess whether your anxiety is caffeine-related. If taking this approach, allow yourself one cup of tea in the morning. Green tea is also full of antioxidants, which we will explore in greater detail in the diet section of this book.

In addition to anxiety, you may suffer from panic attacks. Panic attacks differ from generalized anxiety in that the symptoms are acute, come on quickly, and last for minutes, whereas generalized anxiety can be present for hours, days, weeks, or months. Panic attacks come on suddenly; you may feel terror without warning. These episodes can happen at any time, and you may feel as if you are having a heart attack or are going to die. The fear is an overreaction to the current situation, and you feel out of control.

To deal with anxiety, you may want to use the Relaxation Induction Script (see appendix 1). You can record this script onto an MP3 player or related device and use it when stressed or before using another script or hypnotherapy visualization. This recording will help you develop control over your physical sensations. Training your body to be able to move into a relaxed state through meditation, hypnosis, or self-hypnosis is often an effective defense against panic attacks. This will be discussed further in the hypnosis section. I also offer a recorded relaxation session at the following websites: **http://www.12WeekstoSelfHealing.com** and **http://www.CandessCampbell.com**.

I remember having a panic attack several years ago. I was at Huckleberry's Natural Market, which is a local organic food store. As I checked out, I realized I didn't have my keys. Searching my purse and pockets, I could not find them. My heart began to race, and my breathing became shallow. I then felt as though I could no longer breathe, and the room seemed to be closing in around me. Looking everywhere possible, I then went to my car to find them, without any luck. I was supposed to be on my way to a meditation class and called from a pay phone to leave a message saying that I would be late. If I had been thinking clearly, I would have used my cell phone. I was terrified and it was raining, so I asked a man in the store for a ride to the class, which was about eight blocks away. I could have walked, but I was shaky, scared, and felt as though I could not breathe. In fact, I felt like lying on the grass outside and crying. Just then, I had a flashback to when I was about fourteen years old at a bus stop and had accepted a ride from a man who then abducted me; I ended up in the hospital in a coma. There was a flash of thought that I must have had panic attacks around that time. (I offer more about this incident later.)

When I got to the meditation class, I shared my experience with the group, and they were calm and supportive. I don't remember having had an attack before this incident and have not had a panic attack since. Apparently, the trigger of losing my keys brought up this reaction. Later, I found the keys on the floor of my car between the seat and the door.

Some symptoms of panic attacks include the following:

- "Racing" heart
- Feeling weak, faint, or dizzy
- Tingling or numbness in the hands and fingers
- Sense of terror, impending doom, or death
- Feeling sweaty or having chills
- Chest pains
- Breathing difficulties
- Feeling a loss of control

While panic attacks usually last less than ten minutes, some of the symptoms may linger for a while. Although my panic attack was an isolated incident, people who have had one panic attack tend to then experience them occasionally. If they experience panic attacks often, it's known as panic disorder.

We are not sure of the cause of panic disorder, but changes in life situations can contribute. People who experience anxiety may be more likely to have panic attacks as well. If you suffer from anxiety or panic attacks, please discuss these symptoms with your doctor.

Medication

Given the title of this book, *12 Weeks to Self-Healing*, I will explore different treatments for emotional, acute, and chronic pain, as well as possible treatments for depression and panic disorder. The traditional prescription for pain, depression, and panic disorder has been medication. Physicians are educated about medication and informed that it is most effective when combined with mental health counseling. However, in my experience, few physicians require that the medication be supplemented by counseling.

That being said, medication, meditation, and hypnotherapy have been well researched and documented in terms of acting as effective treatments for emotional, acute, and chronic pain. In this section, I will give an overview of non-medication resources, meditation, and hypnotherapy as methods of addressing pain. A combination of two or more of these may be the ideal choice for you.

I have been combining mental health counseling with energy medicine for over twenty years. In doing so, I've found that there is an emotional basis for most pain. Even with an injury from an accident or other type of physical trauma, the subsequent pain can take on an additional emotional aspect, which may determine how long it takes for the injury to heal.

Most allopathic health care providers will provide medication for pain, as well as for the depression and anxiety relating to it or originating from other issues. Specific pain medications and antidepressants change quickly, so I have not included an overview of those that can be prescribed. Perhaps more importantly, the scope of this book is about *self*-healing and transforming your life through energy medicine. If medication is your choice of treatment once you've read through these pages, I will leave it to your physician to update you on the ones available.

It's important to note that many people do not respond well to medications. I find this to be the case especially with people like myself who are more sensitive to such remedies. Even when I receive alternative treatments like acupuncture, my body responds quickly and balances with little intervention, which is considerably preferable to my experience with medications.

A case to illustrate this point involves my marriage of several years ago, in which the relationship was great as far as connecting intellectually, but my need for physical nurturing and connection was much greater than my husband's need. Over time, I became depressed. My first attempt at a solution was to get a dog. My heart was aching to express and receive love! As much as I adored Friday— the apricot poodle I rescued from the shelter—loving him didn't cure my depression.

In my next attempt at healing, I made an appointment with my physician. He put me on Zoloft, and after a few weeks of adhering to the prescription, I responded badly and was barely able to think. We adjusted the dosage and that didn't help either. Finally, he and I discussed my sensitivity and he referred me to a naturopath, which is a physician who understands and uses integrative medicine. Although my original doctor was open to alternative medicine, I believe the system in which he worked limited his choices around treatment. This is true for so many allopathic doctors today. Luckily my insurance covered my visits with the naturopath.

The naturopath assessed me with adrenal fatigue and prescribed DHEA and licorice to help me. He drew a pie with eight slices and explained that I didn't have to be the one to take care of every part of the pie; I could just do what was my share. He made it clear to me that I was 'overdoing' to the point of compromising my health. It was difficult to see the results of the treatment, primarily because my husband and I divorced not long afterward and I kept pushing myself too hard. However, the treatment lifted my depression, and my mood was good. There are two sides to every story, and what I know from my former husband is that I had a tendency to act as if I knew everything. And, yes, I am a work in progress. Nevertheless, I kept the dog!

I ended up continuing the pattern of 'overdoing' for six more years and again was diagnosed with adrenal fatigue when my energy level became so low that I could barely function. While I talk more about this later in the book, I will say here that I did subsequently follow the help of another naturopath, at which point I found my answer.

You may find that you benefit from pharmaceutical drugs. For those who don't, there are some substance alternatives and behavioral alternatives. Dr. Daniel Amen's book, *Magnificent Mind at Any Age: Natural Ways to Unleash Your Brain's Maximum Potential*, lists seven different types of depression and anxiety, as well as solutions for them all.[5] Here, I will list what he recommends as treatment for all types of depression and anxiety.

First of all, get a physical exam and then begin some type of exercise routine. Exercise boosts the flow of blood and necessary nutrients to the brain, and its effects are comparable to those of antidepressants. Amen reported, "In one head-to-head study comparing exercise with Zoloft, one of our effective antidepressants, they were equally effective after twelve weeks and exercise was actually more effective after ten months."

Next, Amen recommends that patients take a multiple vitamin (multivitamin) and a fish oil supplement daily. He explains that many who are depressed don't eat balanced diets and tend to lack necessary vitamins and minerals, especially Vitamin D. Did you know that you can walk in the sun for twenty minutes a day without sunscreen to make use of your body's own ability to produce Vitamin D? I remember hearing this advice from Dr. Norm Shealy, one of the world's leading experts in pain management, at a workshop. He was also a strong advocate of Vitamin D. Beyond this integral vitamin that many people lack, Dr. Amen also notes that omega-3 fatty acids, which are found in fish oil, have been found to be low in those who suffer from "depression, ADD, Alzheimer's disease, and in those who have suicidal thoughts."

Furthermore, he explains that people with anxiety and depression are often filled with Automatic Negative Thoughts (ANTs). Learning how to correct these negative thought patterns has been found to be as effective as taking antidepressants—and it has no side effects. I will address this concept further in Week Four.

Finally, Amen suggests using natural supplements. He advises trying this approach before taking medication. I suggest you follow the direction of your physician, whichever one you choose to best meet your personal needs, whether allopathic or naturopathic.

Educating yourself about your depression and anxiety is important, and this book provides an overview to guide you in the best direction for self-healing. You may be interested in finding out more about natural supplements, and you may even want to take the Amen Brain System Test online at **http://www.amenclinics.com**.[6]

Another contributor to depression and anxiety is the use of alcohol, marijuana, or other substances. Although this self-medicating may seem to work at first, eventually it will worsen your situation. For most of those who suffer from an addiction, 12-step meetings work the best for most. Check out the local Alcoholics Anonymous, Narcotics Anonymous, Al-Anon, Overeaters Anonymous, or Gamblers Anonymous meeting in your neighborhood (see appendix 9 for resources). Also, if you are abusing alcohol, medication, or other drugs, you can contact your local chemical dependency agency for an evaluation and referral. While some of the techniques in this book will work if you have a problem with any of these substances, you may feel as though you are taking three steps forward and two steps back. Addressing the addiction in conjunction with the information in this book will be extremely helpful.

Body Scan

Before addressing meditation and hypnotherapy, I recommend learning how to use the body scan to identify and assess pain through a pain scale.

When working with pain, it's helpful to be able to identify your *level* of pain. As you use the tools in this book, you will find that the pain moves and changes. This is the gift of self-healing. You will learn to change your pain level and, in many cases, clear the pain altogether. The first step is to practice the body scan. Close your eyes and take a couple of deep breaths. Imagine a grounding cord, such as a rope, tree trunk, or beam of light, starting at the base of your spine and going all the way down to the center of the earth. Consciously release energy, tension, and stress down this grounding cord. Now bring your attention to your scalp. Take notice of any tension, pain, or unusual sensation. Continue moving downward through your body, noticing where you feel the pain. You can use the pain scale to measure the pain. It's helpful to make notes about this in your journal, so you will be able to see how you can change the pain level.

The Comparative Pain Scale

I include the Comparative Pain Scale (Figure 2) to help you determine whether your pain is minor, moderate, or severe. Take a moment to do the assessment. Look at the levels within each group, and select the one that comes closest to describing your level of pain.

	0	No pain. Feeling perfectly normal.
Minor Does not interfere with most activities. Able to adapt to pain psychologically and with medication or devices such as cushions.	1 Very Mild	Very light barely noticeable pain, like a mosquito bite or a poison ivy itch. Most of the time you never think about the pain.
	2 Discomforting	Minor pain, like lightly pinching the fold of skin between the thumb and first finger with the other hand, using the fingernails. Note that people react differently to this self-test.
	3 Tolerable	Very noticeable pain, like an accidental cut, a blow to the nose causing a bloody nose, or a doctor giving you an injection. The pain is not so strong that you cannot get used to it. Eventually, most of the time you don't notice the pain. You have *adapted* to it.
Moderate Interferes with many activities. Requires lifestyle changes but patient remains independent. Unable to adapt to pain.	4 Distressing	Strong, deep pain, like an average toothache, the initial pain from a bee sting, or minor trauma to part of the body, such as stubbing your toe very hard. So strong, you notice the pain all the time and *cannot completely adapt.* This pain level can be simulated by pinching the fold of skin between the thumb and first finger with the other hand, using the fingernails, and squeezing very hard. Note how the simulated pain is initially piercing but becomes dull after that.

	3 Very Distressing	Strong, deep, piercing pain, such as a sprained ankle when you stand on it wrong or mild back pain. Not only do you notice the pain all the time, you are now so preoccupied with managing it that you normal lifestyle is curtailed. Temporary personality disorders are frequent.
	6 Intense	Strong, deep, piercing pain so strong it seems to partially dominate your senses, causing you to think somewhat unclearly. At this point, you begin to have trouble holding a job or maintaining normal social relationships. Comparable to a bad non-migraine headache combined with several bee stings, or a bad back pain.
Severe Unable to engage in normal activities. Patient is disabled and unable to function independently.	7 Very Intense	Same as 6 except the pain completely dominates your senses, causing you to think unclearly about half the time. At this point, you are effectively disabled and frequently cannot live alone. Comparable to an average migraine headache.

Figure 2 Comparative Pain Scale
Comparative Pain Scale from Jack Harich, July 14, 2002. Copyright by Jack Harich. Reprinted with permission.

The Sensory Description of Pain was compiled by Brian E Walsh PhD.[7] This handout is particularly helpful because— in addition to comprehensively describing the sensations—it helps you take note of the level of pain, its frequency, and where you feel it in your body. You can take this handout with you when you see your health care provider in order to communicate clearly and concisely.

SENSORY DESCRIPTION OF PAIN

NAME

Place an **X** to represent the severity of your pain in any category that applies.

	1	2	3	4	5	6	7	8	9	10	Specific Body Location	Frequency
Aching												
Beating												
Binding												
Biting												
Burning												
Caustic												
Cool												
Corroding												
Cramping												
Crushing												
Cutting												
Drilling												
Dull												
Flashing												
Flickering												
Gnawing												
Grinding												
Gripping												
Heavy												
Hot												
Itching												
Lacerating												
Nagging												
Nauseating												
Numb												
Penetrating												
Piercing												
Pinching												
Pounding												

	1	2	3	4	5	6	7	8	9	10	Specific Body Location	Frequency
Pulsing												
Rasping												
Searing												
Sharp												
Shooting												
Smarting												
Spasming												

Figure 3 Sensory Description of Pain

Note: Compiled by author Brian E Walsh PhD. Reprinted with permission.

When working with clients in my office, I have heard over and over that their doctors or other health care providers didn't listen. The Sensory Description of Pain is a great way to bridge this gap of communication, as it will help you to stay focused and describe the facts.

Tools and Exercises

Journaling

There are many reasons to use a journal. You may find that you have an editor working in your mind, even if you're not conscious of it. This internal censor may keep you from expressing (or even being aware of) many of your thoughts. When you write out your thoughts, you are able to get beyond the ego and contact a deeper part of yourself. Your journal can become comforting, like a good friend.

In addition to the free writing described earlier, the following examples are other ways in which you might use your journal:

1. Dear God/Goddess letter – Write a letter to God or Goddess stating everything you need to say. Write as if you are having a private meeting with Him or Her—because you are!

2. Gratitude list – This is one of my favorites. Write down ten things that fill you with gratitude, and eventually work up to a list of twenty. If I find myself in a grumpy mood, I do this daily. It's difficult to be angry or negative after doing so, because this activity seems to lift the heart. Completing this exercise weekly is a great goal to improve your mood.

3. Anger letter – In having journaled for over thirty years, I believe that venting can be quite helpful. When I started going through my journals to pull out the information I wanted to save, I definitely had to sort through the angry letters. Letting this energy go on a piece of paper is much better than turning it inward toward yourself and creating depression or pain—or turning it outward toward a loved one or innocent friend and creating trouble in your relationships.

4. List of to do's – I admit that I am a list person. Writing a list of to do's can prime the pump for action ... especially if you are stuck and need to get moving.

5. Pros/Cons – It's helpful to write out the pros and cons of a situation to get yourself unstuck. Writing this list may turn into a free writing journal entry and help you see what is beneath the indecision.

6. Dreams – When you write down your dreams, you may find that the meaning comes through. To help you in the event you decide to work your dreams, a couple of my favorite books on the topic are as follows: *Realities of the Dreaming Mind: The Practice of Dream Yoga,* by Swami Sivananda Radha, and *Where People Fly and Water Runs Uphill: Using Dreams to Tap the Wisdom of the Unconscious,* by Jeremy Taylor.[8,9] There are many others you might enjoy, and I wish you fun in your search.

7. Poetry/Prose – Creativity often leaves us feeling good about ourselves. A simple poem or prose piece can be a great journal entry. After my father died, I sat on my balcony looking out over the river and wrote a poem that has comforted me for years. The poem is at the end of this section.

8. Notes from books – I love to read, and I often include notes from books in my journal. If it's a nonfiction book, I write the name of the book and keep notes on what I would like to remember and incorporate into my life. With fiction pieces, I often find a method of looking at things anew, or I discover a beautiful way to say something. I make notes of both examples of it in my journal.

9. Inventory of Self – Your journal is a great place to inventory yourself. If you need to be uplifted, write things about yourself that make you feel good. If you are stuck, you might find it useful to write about what you would like to change. I love what Caroline Myss recommended at a workshop I attended. She suggested, "Write out everything you are doing you know you should not be doing and everything you are not doing you know that you should be doing."[10]

10. Priorities – If you are like me, you may find that you can spend a lot of time on insignificant items and get behind on the priorities. Unnecessary details are often distracting. If you find this to be the case, write out your priorities and place them somewhere you often look during the day.

11. Friends – Write down what you love about your friends! Your journal is a wonderful place to change your mood, and this exercise leaves you feeling good. If you have children or grandchildren, you will probably find it fun to write about them as well.

12. Self-love list – Write down what you love about yourself. This is often more difficult to do than some of the others I've described above, but you will find that you can change your mood—and even your life—with this exercise.

This is just a list to get you started; there are plenty of uses and avenues for free writing. I have actually used my journal to take notes at workshops. In doing so, I can go back over my notes and remember the important details from the workshop without reading the handouts or book. Taking the Angel Therapy Practitioner® Class in Kailua-Kona, Hawaii was incredibly fun.[11] When I reread my notes, I found I had made comments about the dolphin swim and snorkeling. Now I can relive the fun times just by looking over the notes I took, which were things that struck me as particularly important in my own process.

My journal took on additional significance when my father died, at which time I looked back in it to where I had written about my mother's death many years before. When you have a loss in the present, the grief from the past attaches to the current loss, and you re-grieve what you lost before as well. Rereading my journal entries about my mother's death helped prepare me for my father's death. I had a blueprint for planning the funeral and settling the estate, and I was better prepared to carry out those steps despite my grief.

As previously mentioned, here is a poem I wrote in my journal during September 2002, after my father died.

Loss

Gazing from the balcony
again this summer
once blessed
by this Spokane River view.
Goldfinch aren't as bright this year
hawks just taunt me with their red tails
circling around my grief.

Blue heron, once majestic,
now indifferent to my pain.
Magpies chide sharply

shaming me at my loss.

Even the river,
once a source of vitality
deep wisdom
forgets to white water wave
as she rolls by.

The fifth summer
once blessed
by this Spokane River view.
This is the year I lost
the year I lost
my dad to cancer
and all the colors
turned to gray.

Support System

Friends

In my private practice, one thing I have noticed is that people who suffer from depression and pain often do not have a support system. A support system is comprised of friends, family, or people who can and will be supportive of you. This may even include a massage therapist, therapist, or acupuncturist.

There was a time when most women worked at home caring for their family, and they created close relationships with their neighbors. They attended neighborhood functions, church activities, and PTA meetings. These people became their support system. Men's friends were often coworkers or the husbands of their wives' friends.

Today, more often than not, women and men are working outside the home, and although they exchange niceties with coworkers, they don't have the intimate, personal conversations that they need in order to heal themselves. Coworkers and business associates may even be competitive and unsupportive. The whole bully attitude has in many cases moved from the playground to the corporate workplace.

Children are no longer available the way they used to be. In today's fast-paced world, they are often too busy for informal, spontaneous, one-to-one social interaction. They connect through texting and by email. Often they move away for one reason or another. People no longer have the kind of access to their children and grandchildren that they once had for support.

When thinking about self-healing, it's important to remember to create friendships that are supportive in nature. Do not spend time or energy on people who are not supportive of you. Notice how you feel after spending time with a friend. Do you feel empowered, or do you find you don't feel good about yourself?

As you age, your awareness moves inward. It's important to continually learn and find things to talk about other than your illnesses. Keep yourself aware of current events. Read novels, watch movies, attend concerts, or find other activities that keep you interested. This allows for better and more varied conversations with friends, family, and your children.

Daily Person

Throughout your lifetime, you will often have what I refer to as a *daily person*. This is a person with whom you speak to "check in" — either daily or several times per week. This person can be your spouse, your child, or a good friend. At this time in my life, my daily person is my close friend named Cheyenne.

In December of 2009, Cheyenne and I were in Japan for a workshop I was facilitating, and I noticed how stressed she became when she was unable to call home. There are few public phones, even in Tokyo, that allow international calls. Eventually she found one, and I have a great picture of her calling home with a big smile when she reached her daughter. Connection with those you love, or your daily person, puts a smile on your face as you share about your day. Whatever the depth of connection you have with your daily person, checking in with him or her near daily is helpful.

If you don't have this type of relationship at this time in your life, create it. When you are not feeling well, although you may talk about your pain, be sure to talk about other topics as well. Also, be sure to ask about your friend and be a good listener. Sometimes your friends can either become overwhelmed by or feel responsible for your health or your mood. It's helpful to let your loved ones know that you just want to share with them. It's also helpful that they understand this is *your* experience, and they are not responsible for your feelings or your health.

There are some friends with whom you can share more details. It helps to journal the deeper feelings first. Then, when you share with a friend, the deeper pain has lessened and the conversation can be more positive.

Have you ever noticed how people match each other's energy? Have you ever been around someone who was angry and noticed later that you felt angry too? What about being around babies or young children? Do you ever notice how you feel uplifted after this experience? The same phenomenon occurs when people are depressed. If you suffer from depression, know that your mood and energy affect those around you. Please note that I am not saying this to make you feel badly about yourself and your feelings. I am saying this for two different reasons altogether. For one, I want you to know that when you're depressed, it's helpful to be around others who are not depressed—primarily if you are in a group of people who are happy, you can begin to feel better by simply being around them. This is where a book club, a quilting class, a historical society meeting, or something else to that effect may help.

The second reason I share this information is that I want you to understand others may not be able to spend as much time with you as you would like. Spend time with those who support you, but do it in short periods such as having a meal together, going for a walk, taking a class, or visiting your local museum. Find activities that are mentally energizing, and be sure to focus on some positive subjects.

Part Two

Moving Into Your Solution

"This is what I hold to be true: belief dictates your life as surely as magnetism directs a compass needle. If you deem yourself unworthy, you'll prove it to be so. If you think you're unfit, you'll find a way to manifest that. I cannot overemphasize both the potential power in our beliefs and the necessity of choosing them wisely."

– Eldon Taylor

Week Two: Finding Your Passion!

After evaluating your situation and discovering more about yourself, the next step is to harness the energy from within to motivate you forward. This is where passion enters.

There seems to be a theme in my counseling and coaching practice. As I listen carefully to the stories of my clients, underneath I continually hear that at some point in their life they gave up their passion. As we explore further, I see more and more that the "should" and "busyness" in life overcame their dreams. Then the emotional and physical pain became present. So, what happened?

Often the busyness of becoming a student, getting a job, getting married, and having children usurped their creativity. They felt lost and didn't know how to become unstuck. They didn't know how to become present to themselves again. This means they became so externally focused that they forgot to simply check in with themselves to see how they were experiencing their life. Somehow, along the line, they forgot to ask themselves if they were happy and what would make them happy. Passion comes from taking time to reflect and living from your excess. When I say, "I see you have lost your passion," they light up, and their answer is, "Yes!"

This week is about regaining your passion. We will focus first on your relationship with yourself and then with the people in your life. We will focus on what supports and what diminishes your efforts to be creative and passionate. We will also look at finding meaning in your life and your life purpose. You will discover how you can identify and create your own passion that carries you beyond the experience of your pain.

What Is Passion?

A good way to explore passion is to think of people you know. Who would you say is passionate? What is it about them that appears to be passionate? What are some characteristics of passion in others? How do you recognize passion in your friends and in yourself? As you think about those who are passionate, ask yourself, "What gives them this special presence?"

Passion is so much more than intense emotion and sensation involving sexuality. In my research, when asking about passion, I've received a number of responses, including, "Passion involves intense feelings, not all of them pleasant." In the same research, inspirational passion has been described as Mother Earth and dance. One woman stated passion for her was the ability to do things she had not been able to do for a bit (due to pain). She noted her pain motivates her to be passionate so that she can continue to play. Others shared they were most passionate when cooking for friends and family. One man responded with a memory of a trip to Nelson, British Columbia that was full of passion for him.

Of course, being a nation of romance, many of us think of falling in love and sensuality when we think of passion. Passion goes much further than this and is the foundation for your increased energy and happiness. What we are exploring here is beyond the amorous look at passion; we are looking at what drives one forward toward a behavior or a goal that brings the person pleasure and happiness. *What makes you feel fully alive?*

Passion can be described as the inner energy that moves you toward creativity, life, love, new adventures, and new ideas with intensity, in order to become more fully who you are and to express yourself wholly and vibrantly in the moment. Passion led me to complete the coursework for my doctorate and then my dissertation, which became this book. I pushed forward, with my nose to the grindstone for three years, even though others doubted I would be able to finish by the university's deadline. This challenge lit me from the inside, and I became very passionate and determined. My passion increased as I gained support from my virtual assistant, my editor, and several friends. It became a team effort and the challenge, support, and passion became contagious.

You will find passion serves you as you focus on your self-healing. It will stir within you a focus and determination to heal and recreate both yourself and your life. When you allow passion to move within, you will notice it shining through you. What's more, you will actually attract others who are passionate as well.

Watch children and you will notice they are full of passion. They are alive, in the moment, and fully expressing themselves. Children are intensely passionate about most of what they think, say, and do. They have an intense desire for knowledge, and they learn easily.

For example, one year I told my tween granddaughter that I would take her to Japan the next time I went to facilitate a seminar. She researched the Internet, found animated shows from Japan, and began to learn about the Japanese culture. I emailed her some photos from my previous trips to Tokyo, Osaka, and Kyoto. Her passion ignited. She decided to learn Japanese, and I bought her a

Japanese language program with games for her Nintendo DS. She immediately began speaking to me in Japanese.

Igniting your passion will move you beyond your normal state of being. Colors are brighter, senses expand, and you move from daily habits to new, exciting ways of experiencing yourself and the world.

I remember the time I was a thirteen-year-old and heard drumming outside my house. It was early evening and, following the sounds, I ended up six blocks away at Franklin Park. There I found the Spokane tribe of American Indians dancing in full regalia, and the park was completely alive with lights. The vibrant dancers and the beat of the drums mesmerized me as I sat and watched for quite some time, captivated by their moves and the colorful clothing, feathers, and jingle dresses. I felt passionate! Today we have access to many cultures on television and the Internet. Notice how they are present in the moment, transformed into another dimension in their creative dance. They are alive and vibrant.

Passion can also mean reconnecting with the inner part of yourself that has gotten lost in the background. I am referencing the part that has taken a backseat to the busyness of your life, as well as your pain.

Let's start by looking within. This may be a difficult challenge for some. Often it is considerably more comfortable to place focus outside yourself, either on another person or on outside situations. I remember driving with some friends one day up to Mount Spokane and back. We were together for several hours. I noticed during the whole trip, not once did anyone share anything about themselves. All the talk was superficial in nature, and there was nothing personal shared whatsoever.

Being the sensitive I am, when we returned, I felt depleted and exhausted. I called another friend, we shared from the heart, and I felt centered again. Passion deals with being in your heart and speaking from your heart. This means feeling vulnerable at times and taking risks. It involves a great deal of focus on understanding yourself and what you need in order to feel passion and that sense of being "centered" — and then fulfilling those needs. In calling a friend with whom I could speak from the heart, I was aware of what I needed and filled that need.

How exactly do you begin to focus on yourself? One method is to begin paying attention to what you do each day. What energizes you, and what makes you feel exhausted? This is about being present to yourself, your thoughts, and your actions. Are you operating throughout your day on automatic pilot?

If so, try changing the order of what you do daily to wake yourself up to your surroundings. Become aware of what you enjoy and what you don't. Sit for a few moments and feel what you feel. What comes up? You may find yourself in a rut, no longer enjoying what you're doing. To be able to move from this state, it is first helpful to become aware of it.

In sitting quietly, feeling your feelings, and allowing yourself to just think about what comes up, you may find that you're experiencing a lot of feelings, but you cannot identify them. A simple way to identify each is to ask yourself whether you feel happy, sad, glad, or mad. Of course, underneath these feelings are variations of them. We will explore this concept in greater detail later.

To illustrate one example now, many people who suffer from pain have a lot of unresolved grief. Grief is a part of sadness that goes underground and often becomes what is known as a low-grade feeling, which is sometimes difficult to identify. You may want to take a moment to think about those whom you have lost in your life, in various ways. Have family members or friends moved away, or have you moved? Have you lost people to death? Have unresolved conflicts caused you to lose touch with folks with whom you were once close? Was there an opportunity you missed in your life? Did you make a choice that left you feeling sad? Did you make one that you regretted later? Did you think your life would turn out differently, and you feel sad about it now? Have you lost some abilities in your body? Is your movement compromised? Is your thinking not as clear as it once was? Does depression keep you from doing what you used to do? Did a traumatic experience ever leave you feeling a sense of loss? I can say from personal experience that I lost almost everything to a house fire in 1987, and that took me a long time to grieve.

All of the above examples offer feelings of grief. We will focus on feeling your feelings in another week, but for now, I want you to use these questions as a way to start identifying the ways in which you have given up following your passion.

Inspired Passion

Earlier, I asked you to identify others you see as passionate. Sometimes we really can ignite our own passions through the example of others. By reading about or identifying with celebrities, authors, dancers, writers, athletes, etc., we are often motivated to create passion. We match their energy and follow what they do to help us manifest our own passion. I know that an example in my own life involves foodie shows. Cooking competitions inspire me to add new ingredients to my limited repertoire of recipes. And, as a writer, I often read something before I begin to write. Consistently reading *Writing a Dissertation in 15 Minutes a Day* for a few minutes before sitting down to write my dissertation was highly motivating and kept me on track.[1]

Commitment

No matter how you are inspired to live passionately, an important facet is commitment. The more you focus on a given subject, the more you become involved. It becomes larger in your life, and you become more intense and encompassed. This often happens with young mothers. Their focus is their children, and they create mothers' groups and congregate with other young mothers. They delight in watching their children and talking about their children, and they glow with passion about being a mom. This passion often spurs them on to write children's books. Grandmothers even often use creativity inspired by their grandchildren to begin a new creative project.

When you think of increasing your passion to support your health, there are many ways to commit. You can educate yourself about your illness and focus on solutions. When you share what you learn with others, this sustains your passion. Helping others who are in a similar situation also strengthens your commitment and passion. Twelve-step groups, such as A.A. (Alcoholics Anonymous) and Al-Anon Family Groups—for friends and family of alcoholics and addicts—are great examples of this. There are many websites where you can share your story, your progress, your motivation, and what you learn about self-healing.

This includes a discussion page that I've organized at **https://www.facebook.com/12WeekstoSelfHealing**.

When you are so committed to your passion, you may sometimes become single-minded. This can be good, or it can narrow and limit your life experience. For instance, if your entire focus is on your illness, you may indeed be passionate about it. But do you just focus on the abilities and joy taken from you? Would it be helpful to focus on solutions as well as creating some distractions from your illness so that you can have a fuller life? Friends are important for support but can become less than fond of hearing the same topic over and over again. Finding several resources and support people can be helpful.

One of the similar pitfalls to being ill is that when you receive a good deal of attention for it, you may shift your own focus so much on your illness that you lose focus on your passions. This is called "secondary gain."

I met a man at a workshop years ago, and we started dating. I had some pain and structural problems in my neck (prior to using a chiropractor), and every time I stretched my neck or rubbed my neck, he immediately gave me a neck rub. With any ache or pain I had, he was overly attentive. I quickly understood that if I continued in this relationship without preventing him from doting on my discomforts, every ache and pain I had would be reinforced. The risk in that was a feeling that my health problems would increase. I loved the attention, but being empowered toward health would have been more supportive.

Think about your life and why you want to be out of pain. If you were not in pain, how would your life be different? Whether you are in situational pain, acute pain, or chronic pain (physical or mental), your feelings can change from day to day. Ask yourself honestly why you want to live. When you think about this, whom is it that you love being around? What is it that you love to do?

You can increase your passion in several areas. In addition to learning about your health and self-healing, focus on activities that balance you in mind, body, emotions, and spirit. For example, you may decide to take a yoga class or a meditation class in which you experience your body, but your mind is not as active. You may instead want to integrate the mind, body, and emotions by taking rock climbing lessons. Perhaps you want to develop your photography skills and explore the incredible nature around you. Laughing while watching a comedy or playing cards or games with friends can also balance you and foster passion!

Passion comes up in many areas of your life. You may be passionate about your family, work, community, politics, creative endeavors, or a class you're taking. My family often meets once or twice a month to play Mexican Dominos or cards. When we travel, we bring back souvenir cards from the cities we visited. We dream about travel and compare our travel experiences. We laugh and are passionate about one another and our time together. Family is often an avenue in which we can express our passion.

Have you ever entered someone's home and noticed it is full of photographs of their family? These people likely delight in showing you the photos of their children and grandchildren. This passion about their family can also expand to passion about photography, framing, or scrapbooking. It also often encompasses hobbies and talents of other family members. If a child is a successful athlete, the mother may experience passion for the sport and the team with which her daughter or son is involved.

Exploring Your Life Purpose

A theme that weaves through exploring passion is finding meaning in your life. As such, one way to expand passion is to identify and explore your life purpose. There are many ways to structure this task. I use the chakra system.

Eastern religions teach that there are seven main chakras in the body; each chakra stores mental, emotional, and spiritual information, and each chakra connects to specific body parts and organs. Awareness of this information assists you in fulfilling your spiritual life lessons—your life purpose. Some people find their purpose early on, and others take a lifetime for it to become clear. Many people mistakenly only focus on their career, but your life purpose encompasses all of your experiences, all of your decisions, and all of your joys. While you will find more information on the chakras in Week Ten and throughout this book, I highlight a bit about each below.

When your life purpose is aligned with the information in the first chakra, the theme of your purpose deals with survival. Your *first chakra* is located near the base of your spine for men and between your ovaries for women. Information in the first chakra involves finding a sense of safety and security for yourself or enabling safety and security for others. You may have issues with your health and find yourself focusing on creating a healthy lifestyle, nurturing others' health, or teaching about health. You may attract experiences where you need to stand up for yourself. You may also find in your life that you often stand up for others. Standing up for yourself or others is a first chakra issue. Many of our greatest leaders have held life purposes connected to the first chakra, and their contribution to the world has come from fulfilling this life purpose.

If your purpose aligns more with *second chakra* information, the issues that you will focus upon in this lifetime are relationships, emotions, intimacy, sexuatity, creativity, work, and money. You will find the second chakra about three inches below your belly button. Explore the relationships that are meaningful to you. To start, look at how you relate to your friends and family. How do these relationships contribute to your emotional and physical health? You may notice that when there is conflict between you and another person, you are in emotional pain or your physical pain increases. You may also notice the opposite is true as well, meaning emotional or physical pain tends to cause conflict between you and others.

Creativity, work, and money are also connected with this chakra and life purpose. Many artists are passionate about their creativity, and it becomes the main focus of their life. We also know many artists who've self-destructed in the pursuit of their passion, so bringing yourself into balance around your life purpose is important. Exploring your life purpose around money can cause a scarcity attitude, which will show up in believing there is not enough money or the feeling that having too much money is wrong. It could also present itself as feeling abundant and attracting money and wealth, no matter your childhood experience. All of this is about bringing yourself into balance around these issues.

If your life purpose is connected with the *third chakra*, it will be important to focus on vitality, energy distribution, inner strength, self-control, power, ego, personality, desire, care of self and others, as well as self-esteem and identity.

The third chakra is located at your solar plexus. You may get a sense in your gut when something happens that does not feel right. You may have a sense that something is wrong or that integrity is lacking. Also, when you respond to something that threatens your ego, you may feel it in your solar plexus, which is your third chakra. With this life purpose, you will have the opportunity to balance your inner strength and self-control with your sense of power and ego. You will have issues that arise around self-care and care of others.

A life purpose set in the third chakra will challenge you to increase your self-esteem and create your unique identity. This may manifest in competitive feelings or feelings of being unworthy. You will find a balance between being easily manipulated or acting like a victim ... and being aggressive, over-functioning, or acting as if you are always right. Once you find this balance, you will have confidence, a great sense of self, and others will listen to you and trust you. This lifetime will be a lot about working on your inner self, balancing yourself, and expressing yourself in a healthy and helpful manner in the world

You probably have a greater sense of the *fourth chakra*— the heart chakra—than any of the others. There is much written and understood about being in your heart. If your life purpose is set in this chakra, the issues you will balance relate to love, self-love, love of others, love of God, affinity, loneliness and commitment, forgiveness and compassion, hope and trust. This is a lifetime of connection with others and, amid difficult situations, learning to keep your heart open. It may also be a lifetime of service to others and giving deeply from your heart.

You may find in this chakra that you vacillate between being extremely loving and being judgmental and critical. You may find you have poor boundaries, that you give and give and give, and that you eventually resent the person you "did so much for" because they "didn't appreciate" you. In this chakra as well as the second, codependency may become an issue. Codependency is when one person focuses more on someone else's life than their own. They generally create a relationship with someone who is addicted or dysfunctional. In my counseling practice, I have seen this thousands of times. Clients who, no matter how many times I redirect them back to themselves, spend the session talking about the other person. In Al-Anon, they say that with a codependent, "When they die, someone else's life flashes before their eyes." This is a serious issue, and I often recommend the book *Codependent No More*, by Melody Beattie.[2]

Developing passion around this life purpose directs you toward deep inner work. Your focus will be about loving yourself, others, and the God of your heart. You will explore compassion, work through feelings of loneliness, and learn about forgiveness. With this as your focus, you have the ability to help others in incredible healing methods.

The *fifth chakra* is located at the throat and relates to communication, choice, strength of will, speech, individual needs, self-expression, and capacity to make decisions. If your life purpose is connected to this information, you may be passionate about communicating your message to the world. You may be a public speaker, teacher, or artist. Perhaps you have a blog. If you are out of balance in this chakra, you could have a weak voice, difficulty speaking up, or you may be overly secretive. On the other end of the spectrum, you could talk excessively, not listen to others, and gossip often. To balance yourself, you will learn to speak directly and honestly. You will listen to others as well as be decisive and open-minded.

The fifth chakra is between the head and the heart. Your life purpose could be about developing a balance between these two chakras. In our society, we often think of men as being "in their head" and women as being "in their heart." A fifth chakra life purpose may be about bringing this balance into the world. I think of writers like John Gray, author of *Men are From Mars and Women are From Venus,* and Gary Chapman, who wrote *The Five Love Languages,* as being examples of this kind of balance between the heart and the head.[3,4] If you find yourself bringing balance to the male and female energies, this may be part of your life purpose.

Your life purpose may be set in the *sixth chakra,* which is located at your brow, between your eyes. The information contained in the sixth chakra relates to insight, clear seeing, clairvoyance, intuition, self-evaluation, intellect, intuition, and wisdom. If this is your passion in this lifetime, you will be balancing yourself in your ability to see clearly, to remember, and to be present to the reality of situations. You may find that in whatever career you choose, you will be developing your intuition and valuing it as much as you value your knowledge. You may choose a spiritual path such as a teacher or an intuitive like myself, or you may use your lifetime to run a corporation or family with intelligence and wisdom.

When you are out of balance in this chakra, you may find that you are insensitive to others, have difficulty visualizing, or have a poor memory. You may have difficulty imagining or remembering your dreams. You may find others saying that you think your way is the only way. Perhaps you are defensive and unable to look at yourself honestly. If this chakra is too open, you may find you have difficulty concentrating or that you have delusions or hallucinations. Your grasp of reality may be limited, or you may come in and out of reality. You may also be obsessive. To bring balance into your life, you must learn to self-evaluate in order to overcome your feelings of inadequacy so that you can focus open-mindedly on your intellect. You will develop congruency between your self-talk and how you feel. You will learn from your mistakes and become aware of how to learn from others' mistakes as well.

The life purpose set in the *seventh chakra* deals with consciousness, knowingness, values, ethics, courage, selflessness, faith and inspiration, as well as spirituality and devotion. This chakra is located a few inches above your head and is like a cone—with the larger area of the cone facing upward and the smaller section closer to your head. With this life purpose, you may find yourself searching and learning excessively about a topic such as religion, politics, or something that deals with values and ethics. You may have strict beliefs you feel compelled to share with others.

Excess in this life purpose may show up as learning difficulties, rigid belief systems, and being overly focused on materialism. You may be cynical of spirituality. On the other side, you may intellectualize and become confused. Friends may say you are in your head too much, or they might ask you to speak in a way they can understand you. They may say you intellectualize or analyze too much. You may be overly focused on spirituality to the point of addiction. You could also develop a devotional practice and become one of the world's leaders in helping others. When you are balanced in this life purpose, you would have the intelligence and wisdom to help others, as well as possess the spiritual desire to do so.

Remember that in learning about all of the chakras as I've described them above, you have taken in a lot of information. The best way for you to understand your life purpose is to read over the descriptions and see what most truly reflects your life. Everyone possesses each of these issues to work through in their lives. Find the one that is most prominent for you. You can find more information about your life purpose and chakras in my upcoming book, *Living Your Life Purpose: Accessing Your Inner Wisdom.*

To summarize, passion is about deep experience. It is about the thoughts and activities that light you up with happiness and lead you toward actions that show your truest self. When you find meaning in your life, your passion increases. Find your life purpose, and—in your own way—live out your passion in being, experiencing, and doing what is most rewarding to you.

Tools and Exercises— "Get out your journal!"

1. When you were an adolescent or younger, about what did you feel passionate? What did you spend your time doing? Who were your friends?

2. In high school, what was your main focus? How did you envision your life would develop? What were your dreams?

3. Who or what inspired you in the past? Who or what inspires you now?

4. Write out a list of people whom you admire. What are their passions as you see them? How do they motivate you to become passionate as well?

5. Do you feel yourself being meaningful to others? Who depends on you the most?

6. Close your eyes and let your mind wander back to times when you felt excited, passionate, and happier than usual. Think about and then journal what you were doing, who was there, what the experience meant to you. Have you done this again? If not, why not?

7. Often we lose our passion with busyness. List some of the ways you distract yourself from doing what you really want to do. What do you tell yourself that distracts you from doing what you love?

8. Another way you may lose your passion is by disconnecting with the voice within. One way I hear people say they do this is by "turning the TV on for white noise." This keeps you from hearing what the soft, inner voice has to say to you! In what ways like this do you tune out your inner voice?

9. Write a list of what you have been grieving. It may be the loss of a person or job, moving from one place to another, or the loss of how you thought your life would be. There are no rules with what you might be grieving. Feel free to be creatively deep.

In healthy relationships, you have room to grow into your best self. You become energized and feel increased by the connection with the other person. For now, let's look at your passionate relationship with yourself. What do you do that increases your passion and your health? It may be taking time to go to the gym, going to a movie with a friend, or even going to the park alone. It may be taking a cooking class, learning how to make sushi, or getting voice lessons. *What is it that you dreamed about when you were younger but never developed in yourself?*

Next, take a look at your relationships with others. Ask yourself these questions:

1. Do I take the time needed to nurture my relationships?

2. Do I ask for what I need or want rather than expect others to read my mind?

3. Do I take the time to plan and follow through with activities and trips necessary to keep a relationship alive?

4. Do I continue to date my loved one rather than fall into a pattern of monotony?

Take some time this month to evaluate what you need to do to become more fully alive, to increase the passion in your life, and to ignite that child part of you that does not resist, but jumps in quickly and playfully ... and grows exponentially!

Week Three: Rule Out and Make Changes
(Diet, Food Intolerance, and Exercise)

Diet

Many books have been written about diets and how to lose weight, and most who follow these suggestions end up in a pattern of yo-yo dieting. Common diets work short-term, and then the sense of deprivation sets in, resulting in a binge.

This section is not about dieting; it is about connecting with your body and learning to listen to what your body needs. It is also about food and healthy food choices. Given the influence of family, friends, and the media—not to mention the prevalence of fad diets—choosing the right foods today can be overwhelming. Even healthy foods can be confusing at times. I will share my story and educate you about some healthy choices. And perhaps most importantly (in my opinion), we will also look at food intolerance, which can also contribute to chronic pain.

If you are having some health or weight issues, I strongly encourage you to contact your health care provider and have some basic tests done. This can rule out illnesses that contribute to your struggle with eating healthy and optimal weight.

Your emotional body is directly related to your eating and health. This reality will be addressed in Week Five on beliefs, as well as in Week Seven on feelings. In the present week, we will explore your relationship with food and your relationship with your body.

Years ago, when I facilitated eating disorder groups and worked with individual clients who were overweight, underweight, or had poor eating habits, I asked them to educate themselves for the first week and not make any changes to their diet other than increasing their water intake and walking. I requested this because often they immediately started dieting, subsequently ate something that didn't fit in with their plan, and by the second meeting they were discouraged. I will ask you as well: please, do not make any changes to your food plan until you finish this week of the process. However, *be sure to increase your water intake*. You may even want to research further before you make any decisions about your food plan otherwise, and I have listed some related resources for you at the end of this book. Also, before you begin a new food plan, I encourage you to consult with your physician or health care provider.

Today, we have access to so many views on health and diet that it can become confusing. In no way am I an expert in this field other than through my own story, which I want to share with you.

I'd like to start by giving some background about growing up in my home. My father was an alcoholic. Although I loved him dearly and he was my main nurturer, he would also binge drink, black out, and behave violently toward my mother. My mother was a good example of the typical victim archetype, and most of the attention she got came from being ill and going to doctors. She had varicose veins removed at age thirty-two. Her first stroke was at age thirty-six, followed by subsequent smaller strokes. She was often ill from pneumonia. When I was a young child, she had what was referred to then as "nervous breakdowns." I imagine today she would be diagnosed with major depressive disorder, recurrent. After suffering from health problems most of her adult life, she died at age fifty-six from cancer directly related to smoking.

What I remember is that when I was a child, my mother was rarely there for me. Because of illness, most of the focus was on her. It seemed from a child's perspective that my mother got her needs met through going to doctors and sharing about her suffering. A common experience for me was sitting at the kitchen table at my grandmother's listening to my mother, grandmother, and two aunts share negatively about their lives and others' lives. The reason I share this is that, in my mind at the time, I decided to stay away from doctors. After all, it seemed my mother's interactions with them replaced her interactions with me.

Nevertheless, as an adult, my energy was significantly decreasing, so I went to a traditional doctor to see if I had fibromyalgia. My thinking was cloudy, I was tired all the time, and my body ached all over. As I was sore wherever he touched, he informed me that he could not test me for fibromyalgia because the diagnosis comes from specific sore points. I left feeling incredibly disappointed.

I then spoke with a friend who was a nurse, asking her what she thought was going on … and she just looked at me. I felt so helpless; she didn't know how to help me either. To solve the problem myself, I joined the gym. Signing up at Curves, I exercised three to five times a week for that entire year. Although this is not the body's normal reaction to exercise, my energy actually decreased, and on some days I could barely move. In my condition, exercising had plummeted me to my bottom.

I later found out I had become so ill that my adrenals didn't function properly, and my body was not digesting food very well. Although I could explain in great detail to my doctor the feeling I had after I ate—a sense of fullness and of my belly expanding while I felt barely able to breathe—I didn't connect that sensation with the inability to digest. I just kept focusing on the fact that I ate less than anyone I knew, and even when I ate two-thirds of what Weight Watchers would allow, I either gained weight or maintained the same weight.

With an office in my home at the time, I was still able to see clients, one of which told me about the naturopath she was seeing for something that sounded similar to what I was experiencing. Ready for a new opportunity that might finally pinpoint the problem, I called Dr. Letitia Dick of the Windrose Naturopathic Clinic in Spokane and made an appointment.[1]

Food Intolerance Test

I reported my symptoms to Dr. Tish (Dr. Letitia Dick-Kronenberg). After speaking with me for a while, she ran the following panel of tests: food intolerance, iridology, microscope analysis, Chapman reflex, deep tendon, Achilles reflex, and the calcium cuff. The one that most fascinated me and offered immediate results was the O.G. Carroll food intolerance test, which looked for digestive or enzyme deficiency issues related to food, rather than immune system allergies. According to Dr. Letitia Dick-Kronenberg, "Since the writing of this, the Washington Department of Licensing is preventing the Carroll test from being performed. A modified version of this food compatibility evaluation is being done at many naturopathic clinics and is in compliance with the current FDA regulations. Hopefully by the time you are reading this, this issue with the Department of Health will be resolved."

To be clear, I had taken either a food allergy or intolerance test in the past, at which time I was given about nine pages of foods that I could and could not eat. I was overwhelmed, put the pages in a file, and went on with my life. The only thing from the list that I remembered was the ability to eat eel. At the time, I was shocked by the thought of eating eel, though I now travel to Japan yearly and happily eat it often.

Rather than having nine pages of foods I could and could not eat, the new food tolerance test gave me two valuable pieces of information. The first was that I have a potato allergy. Although this was a difficult change to make in my diet, my joints stopped aching shortly thereafter, and I was no longer in pain. It was an easy mental switch for me to stop eating potatoes. I have no grief over never having a French fry or mashed potatoes again, but I found that potato is in just about everything! As one of the handouts the doctor gave me advised:

> B Vitamins are cultured from a potato base. The B vitamins (Niacin, Thiamin, and Riboflavin) are used to enrich most baking flours, pasta products, breakfast cereals, and rice. Do not eat any enriched bread or pasta products. The alternative is whole grain pastas from natural food stores and whole wheat flour that you grind yourself or buy to make your own bread.[2]

Potato is also in dextrose (a sugar derivative), iodized salt, baking powder, and so on. You can easily see how this called for a big shift in my eating. Dr. Tish gave me a list of foods I could eat, which included specific brand names that didn't use potato. Additionally, her office completed testing on foods that patients brought in with them. You can find an interactive food list on her website at **http://www.windroseclinic.com/links.html** which has custom food lists specific to your individual food intolerances.[3]

Before seeing Dr. Tish, there were times when I ate and had severe cramps but was unable to figure out the particular food causing the effect. To this end, the second piece of valuable information that I learned from Dr. Tish was my body's inability to process sugar and fruit at the same time. She asked me to try eating these two food items at least eight hours apart, and this suggestion proved incredibly valuable to me. She even recommended attempting to eat sugar one day and fruit the next. My hope is to continue to move away from sugar entirely, but it is a process.

In addition to giving up potato, as well as avoiding eating fruit and sugar within eight hours of each other, I was informed that I should be eating even less than I already consumed. There was a part of me that went into resistance and rationalized with myself upon hearing this news, but the reality is, my body is not someone else's body. If I were to eat the way the average healthy person ate, I could not digest all of the food. Some bodies have difficulty digesting as they get older, and mine is one of them. I finally allowed myself to be kind to my body and eat less. It rewarded me with efficient digestion and the absence of the full, bloated feeling that used to be with me for hours.

There were other suggestions from Dr. Tish, but the main ones were to rest and take the nutritional supplements she prescribed to treat my adrenal fatigue. That year, I filled up my container with the nutritional supplements, took them several times a day as recommended, and I rested. Due to fatigue, some days I could only see one client. There were days I could not walk my dog across the street to the river, and I instead let him out the sliding door into the yard.

Living in a home that was like a detached townhouse, I became fearful and visualized the eventual need to rent the top part of my home and move myself into the lower section of the house, renovating it so that each floor would have its own full bathroom, stove, and refrigerator. I had all but given in and given up after spending months barely able to function.

And then I began to recover. I continued to recover. I did Reiki on myself, which I will talk about further in Week Twelve, and I attended a yoga class in the afternoon occasionally. Over time, I began to feel better and ventured out to listen to local folk music that I love. Then I began wearing a BioPro (now Gia Wellness) pendant that protected me from electromagnetic energy from televisions, computers, microwaves, and other products.[4] This made a big difference in the increase of my energy. I see that the time I spent resting, the change in my diet, the nutritional supplements, and use of healing tools were all incredibly important. In 2008, my business through the Internet took off, and I began to travel more for work, facilitating seminars and taking classes ten days each month for the whole next year.

Cheyenne, my acupuncturist friend mentioned above, explained the results from a Chinese medicinal perspective, saying that my chi was likely deficient many years before I noticed I was ill. What I needed was restorative measures like rest, good nutrition, and reduced stress—not exercise. These are Yin nourishing actions; these were also what Dr. Tish had prescribed.

Regarding your own pain and health, it is vital that you find a physician who knows what is happening in your body and can speak with you about it. Make sure the person is able to give you some solutions to the problem. Medication may be a solution for some but not for others.

Another thing I realize now is that during and after exercise, aside from the little bit of tiredness that comes naturally, I should feel better and energized instead of fully depleted. If exercise depletes you, consider finding an acupuncturist who can take your pulses and diagnose an issue. (In acupuncture, they take twelve pulses—each corresponding to one of your meridians—to see where your body is out of balance.) Also, give yourself the opportunity to journal and self-diagnose some of the issues that are settling in your body as pain. We will discuss this further in subsequent weeks.

The Quality of Food

Once I began to eat less, I also became more interested in the foods I ate. I had heard that eating organic was beneficial, but I never really considered why, so I researched the reason behind eating organic.

Organic Foods

You may notice organic food at your local grocery store. Many wonder the difference between organic broccoli and the broccoli you have been purchasing and eating most of your life. Some of the reasons to eat organic are as follows:

1. Organic foods are safer and have more phytonutrients (nutrients derived from plant

material that have been shown to be necessary for sustaining human life) than non-organic foods.

2. Organic foods taste better!

3. Organic food has more life force. This is the vibration, or energy, of the food. For instance, a fresh apple has more life force than one sitting on your counter for days that begins to wrinkle.

4. Organic food is grown by farmers who are conscious of the importance of renewable resources; this protects the soil and water for future generations.

5. Animals on organic farms are treated better.

6. When the word organic is used in reference to animal products, it means the animals that are the source of those products have not been given growth hormones or antibiotics.

7. Organic food is produced without using pesticides and fertilizers, which may contain synthetic ingredients, sewage sludge, and ionizing radiation.

According to Cheyenne Mendel:

When you look at a non-organic almond farm in California, it looks like a concentration camp. It is all dirt and trees, nothing else. When you look at an organic almond farm, you see a bio-diverse farm with lots of colors, bees, and birds in the trees … In the 50s and 60s corporate farming was supposed to be a solution to end world hunger. We now know, decades later, the devastating side effects of those choices, and it turns out good old fashioned farming methods from over the ages is the way to not only provide food to third world countries, but is the green earth healthy alternative as well.[5]

I remember seeing something on the television last year that showed chickens being genetically altered to have large breasts so we as consumers can have a lot of white breast meat. The chickens are raised in large warehouses, and their beaks are cut off (without anesthesia) so they don't peck each other. With very little room to move, they fall over on each other because their breasts are too big for their little feet to hold them. They are slaughtered at about six weeks. After seeing this, for the most part, I stopped eating chicken. I buy organic chicken when I do eat it, and I always buy free roaming, organic farm eggs.

Although experts are divided on the importance of eating organic food, continuing research supports that eating organic food reduces the amount of toxic chemicals ingested in the body. Organic farms also introduce fewer toxins to the environment.

One particular environmental concern is organophosphates. According to Frances M. Dyro's article entitled "Organophosphates" on the eMedicine website, organophosphates are chemical substances originally produced by the reaction of alcohols and phosphoric acid.[6] These substances were used as insecticides in the 1930s, but the German military developed them as neurotoxins in World War II. Organophosphate insecticides such as diazinon, disulfoton, azinphos-methyl, and fonofos are used widely as pesticides in agricultural and household applications. If you are interested in more information about pesticides and organophosphates, Dr. Mary O'Brien has an interesting report in the *Journal of Pesticide Reform*.[7]

With a little research, you will find that organic foods have more vitamins, minerals, antioxidants, and essential fatty acids due to the quality of soil in which they are grown. Eating organic is more important for some foods than others. If you are slowly moving into organic foods, you may want to begin with buying organic apples, bell peppers, celery, cherries, imported grapes, nectarines, peaches, pears, potatoes, red raspberries, spinach, and strawberries. This is a good list to start, primarily because these foods often retain pesticides even after they've been washed. Remember, organic foods are grown without pesticides.

As Heritage found in the article, "The Fate of Transgenes in the Human Gut," organic foods are also preferable because they are not genetically altered. When our bodies digest genetically modified foods, the character of our intestinal bacteria is altered by the artificially created genes. Heritage and Netherwood, Martin-Orue, O'Donnell, Gockling, Graham et al. note this.[8,9] Moreover, several sources suggest that gene transfer between genetically modified crops and nearby native species has created plants so resistant that they are known as superweeds. Genetic engineers have been criticized as acting without forethought when they introduced genetically modified organisms to unmodified plants. The effects of this oversight are becoming apparent as the genes of the genetically altered plants are altering other plants in turn.[10]

You may wonder what difference exists between organic foods and *certified* organic foods. According to the website of the United States Department of Agriculture, the Organic Foods Production Act (OFPA) and the National Organic

Program (NOP) were enacted and created to monitor and ensure "the organic agricultural products ... are produced, processed, and certified to consistent national organic standards."[11] Operations whose gross income sales for organic food are $5,000 or more annually must have their products certified by USDA-accredited certifying agents. If the sale is less than $5000, they can label the products organic without the certification, but the regulations and standards are the same as for certified organic foods. I understand this can be confusing, so what I do is buy from local stores that I trust, as well as farmer's markets when possible. Also, of course, buying in season gives us the freshest food.

Over the years, I have had friends and clients use a change in diet to heal themselves from cancer and other illnesses. They have done so by eating organic foods and refraining from eating processed foods—foods that come in a bag, box, or can.

This brings up another issue related to food quality, which is the amount of life force left in your food when you eat it. In the section on kinesiology, I will show you how to test the percentage of life force in your food. Foods that are still on the tree, on the bush, or in/on the ground still have all the life force. As such, their nutrient counts are high. Once a fruit or vegetable has been picked, the life force begins to decline. You may have noticed that on some occasions you'll buy an apple that is juicy and tastes exceptionally delicious. On other occasions, you'll buy an apple only to find that it is dry and tasteless with very little juice. When you choose your food, especially if you are limiting your calories, be sure to choose foods with the highest life force.

In addition to packaging, processing, and pesticides, there are many factors that affect the life force of food. One is time. Find food that has been recently picked. Another factor is preparation style. For example, when an apple is juiced or sliced, the life force diminishes. You notice after you peel a banana or cut into an apple that it begins to turn brown. According to Virtue and Prelitz in *Eating in the Light: Making the Switch to Vegetarianism on Your Spiritual Path*, when food is juiced, it keeps its life force for about twenty minutes.[12] She states that additives can also affect the life force of a food. For example, if your foods are full of "preservatives, refined sugar, caffeine, white flour, hormones, and other additives, they have very little life force."[13]

Food also picks up the energy of the animal from which it comes. When you eat the products of an animal, such as milk or meat from a cow that has been in pain, this "can have a negative effect on you, reducing your ability to utilize life-force energy in general."[14] This is why I always buy eggs that are from free-range hens not fed hormones or any other additives. The people handling, cooking, and serving your food can have an effect on it as well. When you eat at restaurants, be sure to choose places where the staff is happy and the chef enjoys cooking the food.

In summation of this section, there are thousands of books full of various diets, some of which you may already have on your bookshelf. Rather than dieting, I recommend the following to assist in healing your body:

1. Get a food intolerance test, preferably one that matches the quality of the O.G. Carroll food intolerance test.[15]

2. Eat organic when you can.

3. Eat local foods.

4. Eat foods that are not processed. This means food that is not boxed, packaged, pre-prepared, or canned.

5. Eat fresh fruits and vegetables that have strong life force.

When you eat a meal, be sure to check in with your body to see how you feel. Are you too full? Does this food give you indigestion? Does it seem to just sit in your stomach? Make note of this feeling so you'll know to avoid that food at a later date. I remember when I was in Kyoto facilitating a workshop in May of 2009. I didn't have access to a stove and subsequently ate out a lot. Sometimes I wasn't sure what I was ordering, and one night I ended up with tempura octopus. It tasted great, but my body would not digest it. The next morning, it felt like the meal was still sitting in my stomach. I now know to understand what my orders actually consist of before I place them.

We will look at this later, but it is important to note here that an element of healthy eating is allowing yourself to receive massage or some other type of nurturing. We are nourished by our food but also need to find ways to be nurtured that don't involve eating. I find making a flavorful tea at night in a special cup or teapot to really help with this. When I was diagnosed with low calcium, my acupuncturist (Cheyenne) shared that one of the best ways to get calcium is through nettle tea, which I found at a local health food store. As it helps increase my calcium *and* offers sedating qualities, nettle tea is a great treat before I go to bed at night.

Exercise

In addition to being bombarded daily with information about the latest diet fads, we are subjected to a lot of changing information about exercise regimens. There are a few things to take into consideration here. First, your pain level and the reason for your pain will definitely affect the style and frequency of your exercising. Having said this, do not let your pain become an excuse or reason to halt you from finding some sort of appropriate exercise plan altogether.

It's my view that the best exercise routine for you is the one that you will do consistently. Think about your personality with respect to motivation and your individual level of stick-to-it-iveness. Maybe you are already exercising on a regular basis, and that is great. It is a lifestyle—one of being fit, which has many rewards.

If you have not developed this habit yet, let's look at a few possible behaviors. Do you start a new exercise plan, buying workout clothes and the latest DVD or new piece of equipment ... and then quit soon after? Do you plan out your activities and keep a journal? Do you post your exercise plan on the refrigerator or a white board and mark off each day you exercise? Are you able to stick to the plan you develop? How do you tell if you've set your expectations too high or too low? Do you then abandon your plan altogether, or do you change your expectations? Do you need a workout partner to inspire you to stick with your exercise plan? How did you determine your plan is not too complicated or unrealistic with your schedule? Are you clear on what you want to accomplish? Maybe you want to feel stronger, lose weight, firm up your body, achieve better motion in your daily movement, fit into your clothes, and/or meet new friends.

You intuitively know more about your body—the best way to get yourself moving and your own particular limitations—than anybody else. I remember friends who were trying to be helpful in encouraging me to do more when my adrenals were shot. I found that I was defending myself and then feeling bad about it. Aside from the short period of rest you may need after activity, exercise should energize you and make you feel better. If you find that not to be the case, please see your physician or health care provider.

And while the above noted intuition is important, it is critical to note that we *all* have physical restrictions and imbalances in our bodies, many of which cause pain. There are movement professionals who can easily and scientifically assess your mobility and stability limitations and imbalances and offer simple, pain-free corrective movements. These correctives often offer immediate and (with practice, as necessary) permanent effects. Chiropractors, physical therapists, yoga/pilates instructors, physical trainers, and medical experts of many other kinds worldwide are learning and espousing Functional Movement Systems (FMS), its screening process, and its corrective strategies.

According to the editor of this book, Pamela Maliniak, who sustained injury from a car accident that doctor after doctor could not diagnose:

> FMS altered my life greatly with respect to pain and my ability to relieve it myself once learning the right tools. Seven years of extreme and often debilitating lower back pain that

radiated throughout my body (caused by a car accident) that was being unsuccessfully or impermanently healed by injections, chiropractic, and what is currently considered conventional physical therapy ... is now gone, and I can control any symptoms that reemerge on my own. I am now able to truly live pain-free and exercise again. What was severely restricted mobility is no longer.[16]

Phil Scarito, FMS and fitness expert specializing in proper, primal, and functional movement, hosts FMS certifications nationwide for fitness and medical professionals looking to learn the craft. On a one-to-one level, he also teaches trainers, doctors, military professionals, and many others from across the globe that understand the need for an effective, non-pill/non-procedure approach to add to traditional approaches—one that doesn't involve perpetual attention and medical visits that act as temporary corrective bandages until the next session. Training these professionals in the proper FMS techniques, he also recommends FMS at the base for all personal training clients before designing any exercise program with his tools of choice: Russian Kettlebells and Indian Clubs. He says:

FMS is a grading system that identifies movement limitations. There are 7 different movements that are tested ... each movement puts the body in different positions, challenging that individual's stability and mobility patterns. These limitations will affect the way someone moves in every way from walking and sitting to running, etc. The entire test only takes 10–12 minutes and should always be administered by an FMS Certified Instructor. If there is pain during the testing of these movements, it is the responsibility of the instructor to refer that client out to a clinician. Pain signals a problem and needs to be assessed, not ignored.[17]

He adds the following:

Everyone who moves can benefit from the FMS screen. We all have limitations in some way. For example, a runner complains of knee pain while running. Usually we relate the pain to age, an old injury, or even old running shoes. Little do we know, we have more control over this than we are taught or aware. The necessary weaknesses and limitations are made evident by the body throughout the FMS screen and can be corrected, with clients often seeing immediate results in change in mobility and/or pain level. Once we have the blueprint to how this person moves, we can then use a very simple algorithm to fix the limitations. Using corrective movements, we can get this person back to a mobile and pain-limited or pain-free life and lower the probability of them becoming injured again in the future. The body wants to heal itself naturally. FMS practitioners, like myself, offer the tools to help it do so.

Please note, as you will with other sections of this book, that FMS practitioners, like members of all professions, offer varying degrees of competence and experience. It is important to check the experience of the practitioner, as well as how often they employ it within their work, looking for one who uses it at the base of their client screening process. If you find a practitioner is not working for you, find another.

In case you do not have a new plan for exercise, or a successful plan from the past on which to draw, I will suggest a few ideas to help you get moving:

1. Find your favorite music—this may even include music to which you loved dancing when you were younger—and begin to dance around your house.

2. When you shop, park farther away and walk to the store. If you are in a parking lot, you can still use the cart to carry your groceries or other purchases back to the car.

3. Explore your neighborhood and walk around the block. Those of us with dogs are often familiar with the areas around our homes. This is a fun way to meet your neighbors and feel a gentle stretch in your body.

4. If you live in extreme weather, either unusually hot or cold, try mall walking. Head there early in the morning, and I propose that you will meet other mall walkers doing the very same thing.

5. Walk in a pool or do water aerobics. This form of exercise is gentle on the body and helps get your heart rate up for health. I often joke that my only sports injury was a blister on my toe from water aerobics.

6. Invest in a bike and ride around your neighborhood. Begin with a short ride and build up your stamina. Others are often eager to join in the fun.

7. Invest in an exercise bike for your home. I have a recumbent bike that I love! I bought a plastic

book-holder for it, and when I read on the bike, an hour simply zooms by. Of course, if an hour seems overwhelming, you might start with five minutes. Most of us can agree to five minutes. If you spend more time on the bike than planned, that is great. If you don't, still pat yourself on the back for accomplishing your five-minute goal.

8. Yoga is generally a good way to strengthen and heal your body. You may want to research the yoga centers around your area. Some have special classes that are healing. One such place is the Radha Yoga Center in my hometown of Spokane, Washington. In addition to Hatha Yoga and other classes, Radha offers a "Yoga of Healing" class and an "Insights from Hatha Yoga" class, in which students reflect on the messages they receive from their body while in the poses.[18] Not all yoga classes are of the same quality, and I encourage you to do some research.

9. Finally, if you are motivated, you can join a gym. Although I pushed myself when I should not have a few years ago, I love working out at Curves. They have a standard half hour workout that raised my heart rate and was attended only by women. If you join a gym and get a professional trainer, make sure you have a trainer who is properly certified and understands your particular needs. Be aware that it is currently an unregulated industry. Although a person may be certified, it does not necessarily mean that he or she is experienced and educated on proper form

and technique to prevent you from pain and injury. There are many types of certifications, so be sure to do your research here as well. If the trainer you choose does not seem to meet your needs—or you experience pain or injury—trust your intuition and try others until you find your fit.

Motivation fluctuates, and it may take time to get to the place you want to be. Do not feel discouraged—enjoy the process of trial and error! You are doing a wonderful thing for yourself and your future. This is one place where it is important to realize that a mishap is not a failure. Instead, it is another step closer to realizing what you will enjoy. Congratulate yourself when that happens! Then reframe your current plan or move on to the next possibility. I find that making continual, small changes works better than making one forceful change that often results in me giving up, but you figure out your own style.

One method I use to start an exercise plan, or to get going again if I let down on my plan, involves engaging a friend's help. When I decided to ride my recumbent bike a half hour each day for a week, I knew I would be motivated by how good I felt. To help myself even further with this goal, I called a girlfriend and told her my plan. I also told her that for every day I didn't accomplish it during the week, I would give her $50. Well, she was delighted, and each time I made up a story in my mind as to why I couldn't ride on a particular day, the $50 kept reappearing right along with the excuse. The result was a great week of exercise! While that was enough to get me going, you can figure out what would keep you from abandoning your plan.

Tools and Exercises

1. Write out a list of foods you eat that you know are not good for you. Now, write out a list of foods that you like that *are* good for you. Allow yourself to increase the foods on the second list and decrease the foods on the first list. This is a process to continue over time; it is not a quick fix.

2. Take a moment and journal about the questions listed in the exercise section of this week. Become clear on what works for you and what does not.

3. Write out your exercise history, including what you have tried in the past, when you did the activity, how long it lasted, and why you stopped. Write out the results from your previous exercise experience.

4. Practice one of the above nine exercise suggestions each day. See how your body feels.

5. Find friends who would also like to change their eating and exercise habits, and make a decision to work together toward your goals.

6. Attend a yoga class once to see if you like it. Yoga is not simply for the body. It is good for the body/mind/spirit.

Remember to reward yourself for positive changes in diet or exercise. I imagine the reduction in your pain will be a reward, but do something fun as well. This might include taking yourself to a movie or buying something you've really wanted.

Week Four: Hypnotherapy

In addition to other methods of self-healing, hypnosis is a valuable tool. This week introduces you to hypnotherapy and self-hypnosis as tools for managing pain and helping you gain control over your life. *Self-Hypnosis, the Complete Manual for Health and Self-Change* is a great resource that has provided much of the information in this week.[1] If you would like further information on using self-hypnosis as a plan to heal your pain, I strongly suggest that you read this book.

Whether you have a session with a hypnotherapist or use self-hypnosis, both are self-healing. I highly suggest finding a hypnotherapist to assist you. Having someone else guide you, witness your experience, and support you is important to healing.

When looking for a hypnotherapist, be aware that it is currently an unregulated industry. Although a person may be certified, it does not necessarily mean that he or she is experienced. Getting referrals from friends or trustworthy associates may be helpful. You can also interview the hypnotherapist to see what his or her training was, how much experience the individual has, and whether or not you feel a sense of rapport. It will be important for you to feel safe with and trust the hypnotherapist you choose.

It's not uncommon to have mixed feelings and beliefs about hypnotherapy. Some people are afraid of being hypnotized. Some think it's a sign of weakness and are sure they cannot be hypnotized. Others associate hypnosis with something entertaining they have seen on television, the Internet, or at a stage show. They think people are controlled and made to do stupid things such as cluck like a chicken.

According to Brian Alman and Peter Lambrou,[2] in stage hypnosis, the stage hypnotherapist carefully screens the volunteers via the questions asked. She may watch the hands that go up after asking the audience, "Who is here to have a good time?" Another question may be, "Who has had a few drinks? Not too many ... just a few?" Again, hands rise excitedly. The hypnotherapist is screening for people who are willing to be lively, fun, and playful—people who are ready to create a funny show. The difference between clinical hypnosis and stage hypnosis is that with clinical hypnosis, the subject focuses on a specific goal. While under clinical hypnosis, people will perform only those behaviors that coincide with their values and their morals. If a suggestion is given that is offensive to the subject in some way, the subject will either ignore the command or come out of hypnosis.

The reality is that you go into and out of trances on a daily basis. It happens often when you are stopped at a red light; your focus drifts, and you don't notice that the light has changed. The person in the car behind you honks the horn, and you are startled back into the present. In this example, you experienced falling into a light trance. You may have also had this experience while washing the dishes, taking a shower, or reading a good book. The telltale sign of having gone into a trance is that you realize you've lost track of time.

This week is about using hypnosis to achieve self-defined goals. In natural trances, your mind goes where it will. With hypnotherapy, you're using the trance to move toward a self-defined goal.

In your first hypnotherapy experience, you may not think you have actually experienced hypnosis, because it feels similar to what you have already experienced as noted in the above paragraph. You are not asleep when in trance, but you are deeply relaxed. If tested, your brain waves would show you to be awake and alert.

While it's not known exactly how hypnosis works, it is helpful to know that the conscious mind is always active. Note that you have a conscious mind and a subconscious mind. Imagine an imaginary line that separates the two. This imaginary line is a protective barrier that keeps the subconscious from popping up into the conscious mind. If you didn't have this separation in your daily life, you would probably have dream-like images floating up from the subconscious. Much as in the dream state, without this imaginary line, it may appear that pigs are flying by while you are walking down the street. When you are in a trance state of hypnosis, this separation is relaxed or disappears, and your whole mind is available to assist you with your goals.

The Lemon Test

You may be wondering if you are a good candidate for hypnosis, and there are a few suggestibility tests used by hypnotherapists to find out. I use the lemon test, which I learned in my certification training from the American Institute of Hypnotherapy in 1999. When the mind is imagining, the body responds as if what it sees is truly occurring. Imagine that you are taking a lemon from the refrigerator. You notice the coolness of the lemon and the bright yellow indentations of the skin. You cut the lemon open, and as the juice sprays your fingers, you see the veins of the lemon and notice its seeds are cut in half. You smell the distinct aroma of citrus in the air and cut the lemon again to make a wedge, exposing more of the juicy fruit. Now, go ahead and pick up the wedge and take a big bite of the lemon …

Did you notice your mouth watering or puckering as you imagined the sourness of the lemon? The body responds as if you had actually taken a bite. My mouth is even watering as I write. This is the power of your mind in creating a physical reality; your body responded as if you had really taken a bite of the lemon, and it will respond when you guide yourself into healing. When you use hypnotherapy for healing, you can create health in your body where illness previously prevailed.

Entering Trance

There are a several ways to enter trance. One is progressive relaxation, and that can be either active or passive. Active progressive relaxation involves tensing the muscles and then relaxing them while practicing breathing. Passive progressive relaxation involves focusing on a part of the body, relaxing through the use of imagery, and releasing tension via the breath.

Eye fixation is another way to enter trance. In this method, you focus on a certain spot—preferably a little above eye level—while giving yourself suggestions to move into trance. You may say, "I feel relaxed and am moving deeper into relaxation." You then allow your eyes to glaze over and slowly close.

You can also use imagery. Imagine a place you have already been or a place you would like to go. You see yourself walking down a path or a stairway. Imagine yourself walking slowly downward. Notice your breath slowing. With each step downward, give yourself suggestions concerning things that you would like to accomplish, or visualize yourself experiencing what you would like to experience.

The more you use hypnotherapy, the more helpful it becomes. Last week, I experienced some anxiety and decided to close my eyes, imagining a ruler that went from 0 to 10. I started with my anxiety at 10, the highest number, and saw the ruler moving down to 0, or no anxiety. As I took a deep breath, my anxiety decreased, and I felt more relaxed.

Music is one of my favorite tools for entering trance. Before you start the music, give yourself suggestions related to how you will respond when it begins. You can also tie the suggestions into the rhythm of the music. For example, when the music is quieter, you may give process suggestions, such as, "My body relaxes with each note." As the music becomes louder, you may give the end result suggestion, such as, "I move easily and have the energy to complete my tasks each day. You can also use a post-hypnotic suggestion, such as, "When I have my tea in the morning, I become pain-free." When you become familiar with a certain piece of music, you're able to orchestrate the self-hypnosis session to the music creatively by allowing the notes to take you deeper and deeper. Sense your breathing as it changes to the rhythm of the music. If this particular technique is not of interest to you, you can choose among many hypnotherapy CDs available on the market to find one that seems right.

To increase your success with self-hypnosis, you may want to practice deepening your trance. This occurs naturally when you put yourself into and out of trance repeatedly. Each time you put yourself in trance again, the trance deepens. You are naturally in trance when you first awaken and right before sleep. These are great times to give yourself suggestions, or to visualize the behavior you would like to accomplish. If movement is difficult for you, you may remain in bed when you awake and image yourself getting up easily. Imagine yourself going through your whole morning routine pain-free and with ease.

Post-Hypnotic Suggestion

When under hypnosis, you can also receive suggestions that you will respond to when you are no longer in a hypnotic state. These are called post-hypnotic cues. They are actions, thoughts, words, images, or events that trigger the post-hypnotic response when you are no longer in trance. For instance, to alleviate acute pain, it's best to prepare yourself with a post-hypnotic suggestion when you are pain-free. While in trance, you may visualize the pain coming on quickly and see yourself drinking a glass of water—as the water is going down your throat, the pain subsides. You may decide to use tensing your fists as the beginning of the cue. Then, when you relax them, the pain subsides. You can use many post-hypnotic cues. Think about what would be natural for you and set that as your cue.

For me, when I visualize petting Domingo, my Cairn Terrier mix, my body relaxes on cue. With chronic pain, the pain level generally ebbs and flows. Prepare your cues when the pain is at the lowest point. With either of these methods, it's important to do it several times in order to achieve the results you want. You can use this with emotional and acute pain as well.

You can also set up a cue to increase your movement or trips to the gym. While in hypnosis, you may sense, feel, and imagine the wonderful feelings you feel after a workout. You imagine the relaxation while in the steam room or the hot tub. You feel the steam on your face and the endorphin high. Then you imagine yourself having a cup of black chai tea in the morning, also feeling the steam on your face. This cue will motivate you to increase your movement or return to the gym. This is just one example, and the choices are infinite. Use your creativity! The more you practice, the easier it will become.

Self-Hypnosis

When you are asleep, you have dreams approximately every ninety minutes. You remember some, while others are immediately forgotten. You have the same dream-like rhythms, called ultradian rhythms, while you are awake. During the daytime, it's important to take a break every ninety minutes or so to rest. Ignoring natural rhythms and pushing through can upset the delicate rhythms of the mind-body regulation. This hyperactivity results in stress-related disorders such as psychosomatic pain, overeating, mood disorders, depression, and other disorders. Honor the natural rhythm of your body. When you find yourself naturally daydreaming or 'spacing out' without seeing, know that unconscious processes are being resolved. This is a vital part of self-healing.

I remember the visit a friend made to my house a few years ago. I proposed heading downtown and listening to music, and she responded that she couldn't go due to feeling tired and needing rest. I was shocked by this response that seemed so foreign to my own reasoning and experience; I had spent years pushing through and doing more, resulting in adrenal fatigue. My friend was connected with her natural need for rest, and hearing her say so eventually changed my life.

When you find yourself pushing through and using caffeine or sugar to keep going, this is the time to listen to your innate ultradian rhythm and take a rest. In fact, you could use the time to initiate a cue. Suggest to yourself that when you move into this natural trance, your body will move into increased self-healing ... and that when you come out of the rhythm, you will be more alert, relaxed, and open to your creative mind.

You may wonder how to tell definitively that you've entered into trance. In *Self-Hypnosis: The Complete Manual for Health and Self-Change* by Alman and Lambrou, the authors explain three clues that allow you to know you've achieved self-hypnosis.[3] One is the experience of relaxation, lower stress levels, and pain reduction. The second is a sensation of warmth, cooling, or numbness during the process. The third hint is a perceived distortion of time. Quite often, the time that has actually passed is much greater than you initially realize. A forty-five minute session can easily feel like five or ten minutes.

When initially practicing self-hypnosis, allowing yourself mini-trances—moving in and out of trance several times a day—is more effective than attempting to experience one session for a longer period of time. You may begin to notice how you naturally move in and out of trance daily. In practicing often, the process of moving into trance intentionally will become quicker, it will feel more familiar, and it will take you less and less time to accomplish your set goal (we will focus on goal setting below).

When you find yourself experiencing self-doubt while in a light trance, focus on the self-doubt and explore the thoughts and feelings underneath it. Allow yourself to become clear about the initial thought that is providing an opening for the self-doubt. Be compassionate toward yourself, and do not judge your thoughts. While this goal may seem daunting, you can accomplish it by committing to a few simple steps. First, as you witness your thought process in this light trance, breathe deeply and focus on your breathing. With each thought, breathe out the self-doubt and then breathe in self-love and confidence. After doing this several times while still in trance, suggest to yourself that whenever self-doubt comes up you will automatically breathe deeply, thus replacing the self-doubt with self-love and feelings of confidence. Making notes about your experience in your journal will be helpful for future sessions.

Goal Setting

In order to begin setting goals, it's critical to become clear on what you want out of your life. Understand that this may not be the same as what others believe to be best for you, including people in your life who offer well-meaning advice. Be sure to set goals that you want and choose, instead of what others want and choose for you.

Although chronic pain is not something anyone would want, there may be benefits to whatever is ailing you. It will be helpful to identify anything related that you might perceive as providing benefit. Once you have done so, it is important to then look at *other* ways in which you can get the same benefits. For example, when you are in pain or become ill, it may be that your children or grandchildren come and visit you more often, and this is a benefit to you. If so, imagine ways in which you could spend time with your family when you are more mobile and not feeling the pain. If the prospect of added affection and attention from family has helped to sustain the pain, finding activities to do with them when you are not in pain would be an appropriate goal.

Other goals may be found by thinking about what you would like to do in your life but have not yet done. Think of all your goals or wishes that have been held back by physical or emotional pain. Which ones would be so meaningful to achieve that you would make a commitment to doing the work necessary to release the pain? We will explore this more in the Tools and Exercises section at the end of this week.

When you want to make a change, often you want it to happen immediately. While it may be possible to reach a goal in one step, remember that it takes many steps to achieve most goals. With larger ones in general, it's quite often better to break up your eventual goal into small steps. This creates small, achievable successes! In forming new behaviors through self-hypnosis, you're also most likely to be successful if you use specific, familiar suggestive images. To maximize effectiveness, allow the steps to build upon each other.

For example, let's say you want to strengthen your body and become more limber. You can begin by imagining yourself as possessing both qualities. In your hypnosis session, you see yourself doing any exercises you choose, though it's helpful to imagine ones with which you are already familiar. If you walk, you may begin seeing yourself walking three days a week. Imagine it step by step, so start by seeing yourself putting on your shoes and getting a drink of water. You might then imagine that you take your MP3 player or cell phone with you. Imagine yourself walking out the door. Sense the bottom of your feet as you step outside. See the houses as you pass by. Smell the trees and flowers. When you use all of your senses, you increase your outcome.

Once you achieve walking three times a week in your literal life, focus on another activity during your hypnotherapy session, such as riding your stationary bike or stretching with a yoga video. Once this goal too has been accomplished in your daily life, you can increase the amount of time you spend walking or doing yoga, or you can increase the frequency of your exercise sessions. You can even start imaging a new exercise in your hypnotherapy sessions. By now, you might even be achieving new exercise goals without using the sessions.

With each step, the unconscious mind becomes the motivation for the next. The conscious mind recognizes the benefits of exercise, such as increased energy and toned muscles, and it increases your motivation. You experience the result you started with by imagining it—the result of feeling stronger and more limber. Your energy level will increase, and your pain will most likely lessen. Remember to start with the exercises you already know or enjoy the most, or begin with those you are positive you will actually carry out. Add the other activities afterward.

Hypnotherapy can be used for so much. Let's say you are having a difficult time with a friend or a family member. While you are alone, you can allow yourself to move into trance and imagine having a conversation with this person. Experience the setting, using all of your senses to set the stage. Feel, smell, and experience the location you're visualizing for this conversation. Imagine the person there before you, and sense in your heart a feeling of love for this person, especially if it has been a difficult relationship. Sense yourself sending them love from your heart. Converse with this person and see them conversing from the heart with you as well. Receive what you would like them to say, and experience a healing and mending of the relationship.

This also works for creating a project or preparing for a test. Whether you have a meeting with a supervisor, a presentation, or a test to take, you can create the scene beforehand and see yourself exactly as you would like to experience the situation. I am sure you have heard of athletes doing this frequently before a big event. You have access to creating at this level as much as you would like.

The list below, which outlines benefits of this approach with respect to healing, is taken from the book entitled *Getting Well Again.*[4]

Setting goals results in the following benefits:

1. Prepares you mentally and emotionally to expect to recover.

2. Allows you to express confidence in your ability to meet your own needs. You become proactive rather than reactive.

3. By working to fulfill your needs, you gain control over your life. This results in a positive self-image.

4. Setting goals helps you to focus your energy. The focus is most effective when it centers on the

process of daily living activities that are attainable. It's ineffective when goals are too difficult and set you up for failure.

Neuro-Linguistic Programming (NLP)

When you create your own suggestions, it's best to put them in the predominant mode of communication that you use. The subconscious is more likely to notice the words or images you use most. In addition, words or images that are familiar may bring with them sensations from a previous experience. These communication modes are called *representational systems* and come from neuro-linguistic programming (NLP).[5] The five types of representational system modes are as follows: visual, auditory, kinesthetic, olfactory, and gustatory. Although we as individuals tend to use all of these, we generally have one or two primary styles. For example, I am predominately kinesthetic. If I were to create an image for relaxing, I would most likely put myself on a beach with the sun shining on my skin. This experience is familiar to me, and my whole body responds immediately with deep breathing, muscle relaxation, and a feeling of the earth supporting my body.

You can figure out your style by thinking about and listening to the words you use in your daily life. Primary visual words include *see*, *look*, *picture*, *show*, and *perspective*. Auditory words include *talk*, *sound*, *hear*, *listen*, *call*, and *tone*. Kinesthetic words include *vibrations*, *soft*, *firm*, *tense*, and *rough*. Olfactory words include *sour*, *smell*, *aroma*, *fragrant*, and *stink*. Gustatory words include *bitter*, *sweet*, *stale*, *salty*, and *taste*.

Here are some examples of these systems, which may help guide you in making your own suggestions. You might find it helpful to use more than one system, and often it's best to use as many senses as you can.

You may use some of the following for pain relief if you are *visually* oriented: as I imagine myself walking down the beach, I *see* the beautiful flowers and *visualize* the many colors. The discomfort I feel in my back turns to *red* like the roses and then changes to *purple* like the iris. As the color changes, the discomfort lessens. I experience the *bright yellow* sunshine coming down through the top of my head, taking all the discomfort with its *shining* light, as it flows down my spine and out the bottom of my feet ...

You may use some of the following for pain relief if you are *auditorily* oriented: I *hear* the *sound* of *bells ringing* from a house nearby, and as the gentle *chimes ring*, the pain dissipates away from my body. This image reminds me of *giggling* with my granddaughter on the patio, where my *chimes ring*. I think of the *cooing sound* of my granddaughter's *voice*, and the pressure in my shoulders fades away.

You may use some of the following for pain relief if you are *kinesthetically* oriented: as I continue on the path, I hear gentle harp music playing. The *vibration* of the music releases the tenseness and pressure in my head. I feel a *cool sense* across my forehead and the intensity lessens. This *coolness* moves to the back of my head and down to my neck as the pain *relaxes* and my whole head *softens* into a *relaxed* state.

You may use some of the following for pain relief if you are *olfactorily* oriented: the *smell* of the beach is *salty*, and I immediately relax as I imagine myself walking in the sand.

The *aroma* of the potted hydrangea relaxes the tension and pain as I recall their *scent* in the garden when I was a child.

You may use some of the following for pain relief if you are **gustatorily** oriented: I sense the *sweetness* of being free from pain, imagining myself feeling this *fresh*, relaxed state throughout the day. My pain level has lessened, and all of these senses will stay with me throughout the day as I continue to move my body without pain.

Again, this is just a sample of how you may create visualization for yourself. You can image this in your mind or even record it and play it for yourself. When creating visualization in any capacity, it is important to eliminate negative statements. Replace any "I should" or "I will not" statements with positive ones, which might include the following: "I see myself," "I will," or "I am."

Stress is one of the strongest factors in illness. Experiencing traumatic situations can cause stress in the body. Less noticeable than traumatic stress is the effect of nonspecific stress that comes from life situations such as work, relationships, financial difficulties, and other everyday events. When dealing with nonspecific stress, it is important to identify the stressors so that you can either avoid them or use your self-hypnosis tool to reduce their effect. The body reacts to stress over time with a fight-or-flight response, which floods the system with adrenaline and other hormones that break down the body's immune system. The weakest part of the body breaks down first. For example, a friend of mine has asthma. Whenever she overstresses herself, her asthma is the signal that she needs to stop and rest.

Self-hypnosis can be helpful with nonspecific stress. Hans Selve used the term *general adaptation syndrome* to describe how the body attempts to deal with nonspecific stress.[6] The three stages include the alarm reaction, a period of resistance, and the exhaustion stage.

For a good example of this, let's look at June. She works in an office, and her cubicle is directly across from that of Lynn, a woman who is more reactive than most to daily situations. Lynn is extremely intense and usually enters a room in an exasperated and hectic manner. After working with Lynn for about a year, whenever June saw, heard, or sensed her, she became alarmed. She quickly moved into resistance. She would feel herself take a short, harsh breath into her throat, and her shoulders and neck would tighten. Lynn typically spent a lot of time on the phone talking loudly, complaining, and being judgmental. When Lynn made a phone call, June knew the reaction soon to follow, and she subsequently became exhausted within minutes.

After June learned self-hypnosis, she employed the strategy whenever she became aware of Lynn. June would surround herself in an imaginary mirror that faced outward, away from herself. This mirror extended two feet above, around, and below her body. June visualized the chaos that Lynn spewed to be quickly reflected back to Lynn. June also imagined that, within the mirrors, she was surrounded with a peaceful and golden light that relaxed her and increased the strength of her immune system. She used a post-hypnotic suggestion to reinforce her self-hypnosis. Whenever June became aware of Lynn and found herself taking short breaths and tightening her shoulders and neck, she would immediately take a deep breath as she touched her right hand to the back of her neck. Instantly, she was surrounded by the golden light. The mirror would surround that, her immune system would strengthen, and she would find her neck and shoulders relaxing effortlessly. After doing this exercise for several sessions, June now finds that she is able to breathe deeply and is no longer in distress when she becomes conscious of Lynn.

Hypnotherapy for Pain Management

Pain is an important cue that can be seen as useful or non-useful. Useful pain alerts you to something negative happening within your body. That is its purpose! It offers you the chance to take action toward healing. Conversely, pain that you've experienced for some time, with origins you already understand, may *not* be useful—unless it reminds you to take it easy and not do more than is healthy for your body. Recognizing your pain symptoms and detailing them allows you to provide information to your medical professional. The reason for the pain must be evaluated before you use hypnosis or self-hypnosis. Prior to beginning, talk with your medical doctor, acupuncturist, or health care professional to make sure the symptom is not related to an illness that needs medical treatment.

Chronic pain is a sign of tissue damage. Once it has been determined whether pain is useful or non-useful, you can use self-hypnosis or hypnosis to control it. By being selective, focusing on a specific area, and allowing for awareness to any change in sensation, you can become conscious of a new problem or a change in symptoms.

It's true that hypnosis can often alleviate unwanted pain and result in you no longer needing related pain medication. Victor Rusch, a dental surgeon who was experienced with hypnosis and self-hypnosis, used self-hypnosis as his only form of anesthesia when having his gallbladder removed.[7] This was an unusual case but nevertheless remarkable. Your experience with self-hypnosis will more likely be intended to manage pain from migraines, back discomfort of all levels, arthritis, or other illnesses and injuries.

Change in pain depends on the person, level of pain, how long he or she has experienced it, and other variables. I find that those who believe they can change their pain level or even heal through their own beliefs and self-hypnosis obtain results more quickly than those who do not.

In *Getting Well Again*, the authors use pain as a sort of biofeedback tool.[8] Their program offers help to cancer patients, but the tools are helpful for those who have other types of pain as well. As the authors explain, "Pain, or the absence of pain becomes a communication from the body about the various activities patients may be engaged in, or the thoughts or problems they may be working on mentally."[9] Often, the onset of pain is linked to an event or a person, so it is important to notice what you are thinking as the pain appears. Building a relationship with your pain can be helpful, and in the Tools and Exercises section to follow, I have created a few exercises for noticing and managing your pain in a new way.

You may want to try a few of the many self-hypnosis techniques I offer in this week to find the one that is best for you. Consider which you are most likely to implement. Also, notice your response to the processes. Do you enjoy listening to music more than progressive relaxation? Take note of how quickly the pain subsides and how long it is managed with one technique versus another. Using a journal will be helpful in keeping track of each technique's effectiveness, in addition to the many other journal functions I described in Week One.

In my career as a mental health therapist, hypnotherapist, and chemical dependency counselor, I often encounter clients whose pain has not been useful in helping them assess whether or not there is something more severe happening in their bodies. Instead, the pain has proven itself useful for other reasons. For instance, if they do not want to go back to work, the pain allows them to stay home or on extended sick leave or disability. Sometimes they continue to experience the pain because the sympathy they receive is comforting and makes them feel important and cared for— and sometimes it is even to make someone else feel guilty or responsible. This is called *secondary gain*. This sort of situation may be difficult for you to honestly assess, especially if someone else gave you this book to read and work through, and you are not motivated to read it on your own. Please take the time to inventory yourself and think if there might be any truth to it in your own situation. I am not judging you in asking, and neither should you be judging yourself. Instead, consider it a potentially groundbreaking foundational step in your healing. What would you be doing now if you were completely healthy? What might you lose if you were healthy and pain free? Do you believe the people who give you attention for being in pain will not offer you attention when you are out of pain? As Mark Twain once said, "There is no large trial without some small compensation." What compensation do you receive as a result of your pain?

I remember a client who was suffering from chronic pain. She found herself resistant to doing the emotional work she needed to in order to let go of the pain. As we looked more closely at her situation, it became clear to her that if she were to be healthy, she would have to leave her current relationship. The man in her life at the time was a benefit to her because he took care of her. She realized that if she were able to care for herself, she would not be as attracted to him and would not need him. She feared the relationship would end, and this fear of change kept her ill for many years.

As you learn to manage your pain through hypnosis, self-hypnosis, and otherwise, be aware that you can choose to eliminate specific pain while continuing to experience sensations that are necessary in alerting you to other health dangers. As Alman and Lambrou explain, "Pain is not an external sensation. We create the feeling of pain in our brains. It serves our survival needs and we have the ultimate control over it."[10]

Chronic pain sufferers usually have a history of going to doctors and other medical practitioners in addition to trying medication and other treatments, to no avail. The resulting sense of helplessness can create other problems such as depression, relationship issues, loss of job, loss of movement, weight gain, and more. Hypnosis can be used to treat all of these issues. Healing through hypnosis is rarely instantaneous. Usually it takes time, but it does work, offering you a way to take control of your life again. This book is just the beginning. I have provided many resources for you to continue with your healing once you are finished here.

Hypnosis Regression

In addition to using self-hypnosis for self-healing, many find it helpful to contact a hypnotherapist or use hypnotherapy CDs. Throughout this process, you may find that your present illness is connected to a past life.

There are many different theories about past lives, even among those who believe in reincarnation. Some believe that you actually live lifetime after lifetime learning lessons and developing your soul. Others believe that you connect to what Carl Jung (1875-1961), a Swiss psychiatrist whose work emphasized our longing for the transcendent, referred to as the *collective unconscious*—a universal repository of all religious, spiritual, and mythological symbols and experiences.[11] The idea is that as you tap into this collective unconscious, you sense information. This explains why many people believe they once lived as Cleopatra or another famous person. Einstein said, "Men invented time to feel comfortable in space. But it doesn't actually exist. All experience is happening at once."

Have you ever felt as if you have lived somewhere that you've never been before? Do you have an affinity for Greece or Italy? Do you find that you read voraciously about a certain place or time in history? Do you squirm when a certain historic event is reenacted on a movie screen? Pay attention to your intuition and allow yourself to open to possibilities of past lives.

For me, it's not important what the truth is about how we connect with this past life information. What is important is the healing. Often the past life regression alone releases the pain. Other clients find comfort because they come to understand why they have the pain, and they continue with hypnosis and other alternative and medical treatments.

Relaxation and Imagery

This week has focused on several aspects of hypnotherapy. In general, there is great value in using hypnotherapy for relaxation and mental imagery to shape your life. According to *Getting Well Again*, the main benefit of relaxation and mental imagery is to break the cycle of tension and fear.[12] This shift increases the patient's ability to have a more positive perspective and increased energy, which helps them to believe and understand that recovery is possible. Biofeedback researchers are demonstrating that relaxation and mental imagery allow people to control inner psychological states, as well as their resulting heart rate, blood pressure, and skin temperature.[13] Simonton cites Barbara Brown, a pioneer in biofeedback research, as explaining:

> If some medical researchers are now teaching hearts, or the minds of hearts, to reverse a pathological condition, then medicine must be learning that relationships between mind and body are more powerful than they thought. The concept of "psychosomatic" is generally accepted as indicating the mental origin of physical pathology; research into biofeedback is the first medically testable indication that the mind can relieve illnesses as well as create them. [Emphasis Simonton's][14]

This can alleviate the need for medications that could be dangerous and expensive. *Getting Well Again* explains that doing the exercises will result in the following benefits:[15]

1. Reduce fear by offering a sense of control.

2. Strengthen the will to live through change in attitude.

3. Effect physical changes such as increasing the immune system and altering the course of malignancy.

4. Assist in evaluating and altering beliefs.

5. Assist in communicating with the unconscious where many beliefs are partially buried.

6. Decrease tension and stress.

7. Move one from hopelessness and helplessness to confidence and optimism.

To assist with your healing, I provide hypnotherapy sessions that you can download to your MP3 player, as well as a relaxation session, a hypnotherapy session for pain, and a smoking cessation hypnotherapy session (along with an audio recording about nutritional support and some journal questions to help you stop smoking). You will find these and much more at **http://www.12WeekstoSelfHealing.com** and **http://www .CandessCampbell.com**.

Tools and Exercises

1. Develop a mantra. A mantra is a short phrase that has an easy rhythm and is used to increase results in your healing process. For example, a mantra in the early morning might be, "I am alive, awake, refreshed, and protected from stress." My favorite walking mantra is, "I am strong, healthy, and fit." An evening mantra might be, "Thank you for my blessings, and heal me in my sleep." There is more about mantras in Week Eight on prayer and meditation. Take a moment to write a mantra in

your journal that you can use in the daytime to support your self-hypnosis experience.

2. Practice writing self-hypnosis suggestions. Decide what you would like to accomplish in this script. Your goal may be to decrease stress, reduce pain, increase exercise, eat a healthy diet, or any number of other life improvements. Write out your suggestions, such as the following: "I crave healthy foods such as green, fresh spinach salad and juicy, organic oranges," "When I feel hungry, I check to see if I am actually thirsty for water instead," and "When I awake, I get out of bed and begin stretching gently."

3. Write in your journal one or more examples of what you would love to do in your life but have not yet done.

What would you want to do so much that you would fight to release your pain in order to have this experience? Make sure these goals have personal meaning for you and that you are not achieving them for someone else. Make sure they will bring you pleasure. Check the goals to see that they are concrete, specific, measurable, and realistic. Put yourself into a light trance and use mental imagery to visualize these goals throughout the day.

4. Download the Pain Management Hypnotherapy Session from my website, practice it daily, and keep a log of your pain in your journal.

5. Use the Comparative Pain Scale found in Week One to chronicle your pain. Write down the time the pain began and what was happening, as well as what you were thinking at the time. Write down the duration of the pain and your response to it. Some healing responses are as follows:

a) Notice the pain. Focus your attention on it, and observe how it changes.

b) Imagine the pain as a color, a shape, and a size. Now change the color, then change the shape, and then change the size. Manipulate the image of the pain. Move it close, move it far away, lighten the color, darken the color, change it to black and white, and eventually have it disappear. This is an NLP technique. NLP is a method described earlier in this week.

c) Communicate with the pain. Ask it what it needs, why it has chosen to come to you, and what you can do to help it go away. Talk to the part of your body that houses the pain. Communicate as if you were getting to know the pain. You can do this in a light trance, or you can put yourself in a light trance and use automatic writing as described in the first week.

6. In your journal, identify and list several benefits you may be receiving from your illness. If it feels safe, you may want to ask friends and family to assist you in this brainstorming process. Examples may be having permission to work less or spend more time at home, having more time to write, sew, or golf—whatever you enjoy. After you have an extensive list, put a star by the five benefits that are most important to you.

Next, review your list. Assess the underlying needs that are met by your illness. You may use the four basic needs William Glasser describes in his book entitled *Choice Theory*.[16] Though we've already discussed this, it is worth mentioning again. He explains that humans behave the best they can at any given time in order to meet one of the four basic needs. These needs are for (1) power and worth, (2) love and belonging, (3) freedom, and (4) fun. Glasser asserts that the majority of human behavior is intended to meet one of these four needs. You may be able to identify this need for yourself quickly, or you may need to ponder it awhile.

As you look at the benefits of your illness, note and pay careful attention to any of the benefits that leave you feeling particularly uncomfortable.

Sometimes emotional discomfort can be a clue to a deeper process. For example, you may find that you get attention from your daughter when you are in pain because she comes to visit and attend to your needs. This could have begun after a surgery or an accident, and you find you don't want to let her know you feel better because you don't want her to stop coming to see you on a regular basis. The benefit of your pain would feed your need for love and belonging.

7. You can also heal through trance. Identify the beliefs and rules that keep you from getting your needs met. Take the example of a woman whose desire is to work part-time and garden, but whose self-esteem is tied directly to performing and achieving professionally. This attitude comes from her family's work ethic expectation. Another example may be a man who wants to buy a home and have a family but instead enlists in the military because his father and grandfather were both officers and military service is expected of him.

8. For another example of healing through trance, list places that have always attracted or repelled you for no known reason. List historical events with which you feel a resonance and those which you distinctly prefer to avoid. Close your eyes and allow yourself to drift into trance. You may

want to use music to assist you with this deepening. See yourself floating backward to a time and place that has a direct connection with your body pain today. See yourself there. Look down at your feet and see what you are wearing on your feet. Look upward to your clothing. What are you wearing? Are you male or female? Are you sitting or standing? Do you have anything in your hands? Are you wearing a belt? Holding a purse? What do they look like? Look around. Do you see people or buildings? What is happening? Get a sense of the time based on what you see. This is just a sample of a past life reading. If you sense that this experience will bring up too much emotion, it will be better for you to find a local hypnotherapist to take you through the process. You can come out of trance by just opening your eyes and saying "I am fully awake." Sit and be sure you are awake before you move around the room.

Another way to access a past life is through automatic writing. Set the intention that a past life will come through. Put yourself in a light trance, pick up a pen, and follow what comes through when you write. You may want to try this a few times to get the full experience. Trust what you get!

Week Five: Assess Your Beliefs

You can think about beliefs in many ways. They are attitudes, viewpoints, ideas, thoughts, values, perceptions, and more. Over the years, I have learned not to share too much about my beliefs in general conversation with those who only challenge and argue. However, I do appreciate hearing the beliefs of others. I understand that each of us gets only a glimpse of *the truth*.

I attended a certification class taught by The Earthstewards Network (**http://www.earthstewards.org**) in the 1990s.[1] This certification allows me to facilitate the workshop entitled Essential Peacemaking: Women and Men, a one-day workshop that brings men and women together in communication. One of the sessions covers the Truth Box and collaborative sharing, which offers a great example of perception. Three sides of the box have a hole. During the workshop, we insist that the content of the box is the *Absolute Truth!* Each person looks into a hole to find the truth, and inside the box are three different pictures. One person looks in and sees a beautiful mountain. Another sees a warm beach, and the third sees the picture of a gorilla. Each person is encouraged to defend their perception and find others who agree. Each picture is the truth, but not the whole truth. This exercise, coupled with the processes of the whole day, help participants to open their minds to the perceptions of others.

We all have only a slice of *the truth*. This is our perception, upon which we build our beliefs. As a therapist, I have been honored to hear the beliefs of many people and learn how their lives are intertwined with their beliefs. If I think it will be helpful to the client, I share my own beliefs. I do not do this often though, as my main goal is to create safety. *In order to heal, we need to feel safe.* When we challenge another's belief, often that person does not feel safe. This is why a gentle expansion of belief can be helpful. My hope is that this book will gently open you to the belief that—yes—you can heal!

Another foundational belief presented in this book is that physical illness has its origin in beliefs, and beliefs create emotional responses. When I assess a client to create a treatment plan, I focus on the person's history, the stories they tell themselves about the past, and their emotional response to those stories. When a client comes in with a physical ailment, more often than not, the pain changes or goes away due to the use of the tools provided in this book. Pain, like emotion, comes and goes. When the pain returns, these tools provide the opportunity for people to impact their lives in a healing way.

Part of the inspiration for this book comes from working with a client who came to me directly from the psychiatric ward at a local hospital. She had been suicidal and was severely depressed. After doing the intake, I encouraged her to buy and work through a book called *The Artist's Way: A Spiritual Path to Higher Creativity*, written by Julia Cameron.[2] Over several weeks, as the client read and completed the exercises in the book, I watched her transform into a lively, hopeful, spirited woman who was ready to continue her life and work. She had a history of sexual abuse by a family member, as well as a mother whom she described as being extremely controlling and suffering from rheumatoid arthritis. The client suffered from rheumatoid arthritis as well, and with her stress, she was beginning to feel pain in her joints. Over the course of several weeks, I witnessed her process. She was happy and became able to discontinue the use of antidepressants. Although she had expected to follow in her mother's path with arthritis, she was doing well and feeling no pain.

In the subsequent few weeks, stress at work and the continued pressure applied by her mother seemed to be more than she could handle. The depression and rheumatoid arthritis reappeared, and the client became suicidal again. It amazed me to watch her transform back into the depressed woman I had first met as she shared with me what she was experiencing at work and in her relationship with her mother. Her mother, crippled with arthritis, continually saw the worst-case scenario and was negative and discouraging. She fed my client's worst fear—that she would become crippled as well.

I attempted to support her and lead her back into health, but her environment was such that it appeared she just got lost in the fear and negativity. She quickly declined, lost her ability to work, and ended up in the hospital again in suicidal despair. Soon she was on disability and was no longer able to meet with me.

I was shocked by this client's quick deterioration and, to be honest, a little fearful myself. My mother had suffered her first stroke at age thirty-six and experienced several afterward. She was often in pain, negative, and helpless. In the end, she died quickly of cancer at age fifty-six, which was a direct result of smoking cigarettes. I had it in the back of my mind that I would live past my mother's age. In these years approaching age fifty-six, I work as much magic as I can to remember that I am not my mother, and my body is not hers. I understand that our beliefs control our health much more than our genetics do, which is a belief that seemed to me to be clearly (although sadly) evidenced by my client's case. I was delighted to find this very belief outlined so clearly by Bruce Lipton in *Biology of Belief*.[3]

Lipton is a medical doctor and scientist whose main study has been cell biology. He asserts the following:

> The world is filled with people who live in constant fear that, on some unsuspecting day, their genes are going to turn on them. Consider the masses of people who think they are ticking time bombs; they wait for cancer to explode in their lives as it exploded in the life of their mother or brother or sister or aunt or uncle. Millions of others attribute their failing health not to a combination of mental, physical, emotional, and spiritual causes, but simply to the inadequacies of their body's biochemical mechanics. ... But single-gene disorders affect less than two percent of the population; the vast majority of people come into this world with genes that should enable them to live a happy and healthy life.[4]

Lipton explains that genes are not activated until they are triggered. What triggers a gene? He references Nijhout's 1990 article called "Metaphors and the Role of Genes in Development" for the answer—the environment! Nijhout explains, "When a gene product is needed a signal from its environment, not an emergent property of the gene itself, activates the expression of that gene."[5] In the case of my client, I would go further to say that her genes were triggered by experiences with childhood sexual abuse, as well as her job, mother, divorce, joint pain, and—more importantly—what she believed, including the stories she told herself about all of it. I say this not to express a lack of compassion for her situation, but to verify that we do have a choice about our health.

At the same time, it is important not to fall into the belief that we are responsible for our illness or begin to blame ourselves. We are all in process, and the learning curve is steep as we pull away from the mainstream beliefs and move toward self-healing. Part of self-healing is having compassion for ourselves where we are right now.

As far as my own health and strokes, I am cautious and eat well. The carotid artery stroke screening I had last week assessed me as being in the normal range, and I have surpassed my mother's age. Nevertheless, about a month ago I set up an appointment to get medical insurance at the urging of my brother. I met with a kind man who explained the programs to me and said, "Okay, you have twelve years until you can retire." I went blank and simply looked at him. Never in my mind had I thought of retirement, and it hadn't occurred to me that I would be sixty-five years old in twelve years. I went home and shook my friend Julie and my brother as I implored, "Why didn't you tell me I was old! I had no idea!"

They laughed, since they had both talked to me about medical insurance for years, and replied, "We did tell you! You wouldn't listen!" (I'm convinced that being consciously *unaware* of my age in relationship to the retirement age has actually kept my arteries clear and my blood pressure down.)

On a more serious note, sometimes our experiences offer a deeper awareness into beliefs we may not even realize we've carried through life. In September of 2008, I made an interesting trip to Nashville, Tennessee to facilitate a spiritual workshop. I went there also planning to spend as much time as possible in the honky-tonks, listening to the music that has nurtured me for years. When I was a child, my dad and I went on weekend trips to the horse races all around Washington and Idaho, and we joined in with the sing-alongs on the radio. Today, I have several friends in Spokane who are musicians, and I love to listen to folk, blues, soft rock, and country music. Music is very nurturing to me.

As soon as I arrived in Nashville, I fell in love with the feeling of its energy. I drove to Brentwood, a suburb of Nashville, and spent several days with my new friends and hosts in their lovely home. It was a townhouse set up against a wilderness area, and their deck was adjacent to trees full of birds and a nearby spring. The home was light, fresh, and airy, and it had very little technology, which was unlike my home that is still saturated with electronics. It was so delightfully peaceful there, partially also due to their personal energy that was also light and gentle. I imagine this came from the fact that they meditated for at least an hour a day.

While there, I traveled into downtown Nashville to facilitate my workshop and private client sessions. The workshop was held at a clinic that was also light and airy. I sensed an amazing attitude of abundance in the people of Nashville, and I felt it from everyone. There is affluence there, but there is an attitude of abundance as well. It is one of openness, receiving, and tremendous giving. The trip turned out to be financially successful for me in a new way as I was able to make an abundance of money while there. Previously when I had traveled, I made contacts for later phone sessions, but I often lost money in the process.

When I returned home, I wanted to share my excitement about the trip and abundance with friends and family. However, I found I couldn't talk about it. I searched my mind and realized that I didn't feel safe sharing this success. It felt overwhelming, and I imagined seeing either disbelief or judgment in the faces of my loved ones. I felt overloaded when I returned home, because I had been intensely attentive to others and my body hurt. Caring for others, traveling across the country, and dealing with my own internal process around changes in my business had left me vulnerable and depleted.

I realized the extent to which the experience of my hometown, Spokane, has been about poverty. My own childhood was financially difficult, given that my father suffered from alcoholism and gambled. As a young woman, I was a single mom struggling to feed two daughters. I wondered why I personally continued to see poverty as a large part of Spokane. I live in Peaceful Valley, a mixed area of small, quaint, historic houses that may have up to 1000 square feet, interspersed with new homes ranging in value from $100,000 to $1,000,000.

I realized how affected I was by the beliefs I had been taught as a child. When I was a little girl, I would often sit at the table with the matriarchs of the family: my mom, my aunts, and my grandmother. One belief I heard repeatedly was that when you have a lot of money, you are not as godly. The women in my family, having struggled financially and in many other ways in their lives, were adamantly critical of others. Their beliefs were grounded with Bible verses. I remember hearing time and again, "It is easier for a camel to go through the eye of a needle than it is for a rich man to enter the kingdom of heaven" (Matthew 19:24). No wonder I didn't feel safe in sharing about my success with family.

Over the years, based on metaphysical readings and my training as a mental health therapist, I have come to believe that our response to life is based on our beliefs. It holds the power in terms of what happens to us. Having come from the belief system in which I was raised, I followed my family's example and struggled financially but never did take on the negativity. I found as much enjoyment and hope in mopping floors at a nursing home when I was nineteen years old as I did as the clinical director of an inpatient/outpatient chemical dependency treatment center later in life.

My Nashville experience inspired me to inventory my beliefs about money and my own personal worth. This pondering resulted in my recording a CD about creating abundance. I believe there is abundance in the world. I believe that as I create abundance for myself, I am more able to joyfully share. My hope is to share with you, motivate you, and inspire you to allow abundance to enter your life. My wish is for you to find abundance in good health, friends, interests, happiness, and finances.

Your attitude toward health and commitment to being present to yourself is a process of becoming. Many people in the United States and other countries tend to externalize their life. They surround themselves with possessions and present themselves in terms of their clothes, the jewelry they wear, and the car they drive. These things become who they are. However, in the process of becoming, you will begin to focus more within. You will begin to learn who you are by listening to your thoughts, examining your choices, developing your intuition, and accessing your passion and creativity. Once this happens, you will continue to express yourself in the world, but those expressions will be a glimpse into who you are, rather than a distraction from the self.

In the first week, I introduced meditation and journaling as methods you can use to move inward and experience your own inner quality. Next, we will explore connecting with your inner wisdom.

How to Develop Your Intuition

Many people have asked me how I became clairvoyant. It was not until I began teaching a class on clairvoyance in 1999 that I realized we are all clairvoyant as children. You tend to lose this ability as a child when you are teased or if you do not have someone to validate it. Your family is usually the cause of giving up intuitive ability, but peer pressure can be a cause as well.

I have a young granddaughter who is clairvoyant, and I support her abilities. I encourage her to write about her experiences, especially since she has an incredible writing ability. She told me she couldn't write because she would lose her friends. Even when I suggested using a pen name, she was still indoctrinated in the belief that it is not okay to have this gift. It is safer for her to not stand out as being different and only share experiences that are similar to those of her friends. At her age, wanting to be like friends is age-appropriate. Because of this, I take her to festivals such as the Fairy Congress in Twisp, Washington.[6] This in an annual event in the North Central Cascades, where hundreds of people attend workshops, dance, and play in celebration of nature spirits, devas, and the faery realms.

When I teach classes, it becomes apparent that when the students share with each other, they remember many incidents of clairvoyance from childhood. This happens because they are in a safe environment in which clairvoyance is acceptable. In addition, as they learn more about what intuition really is, they recognize how intuitive they really are.

In this week, I will help you identify and expand your own clairvoyant ability, as each person has an individualized primary way of getting information. In Week

Three, we looked at neuro-linguistic programming and the representational modes. You began to understand the primary methods of experiencing, which included visual, auditory, kinesthetic, olfactory, and gustatory. A simple list of words for each system is included in appendix 2. This is the NLP Word List. As you begin to develop your clairvoyance, you may want to study these words to assist you in getting clear and detailed information.

The representational system uses the five senses to identify how you organize your experiences. When developing your clairvoyance, you use four primary ways of getting information. They are clairsentience (clear-feeling), claircognizance (clear-knowing), clairaudience (clear-hearing), and clairvoyance (clear-seeing).

Because my clairvoyant ability comes to me naturally, it is difficult to explain it to others. I am happy that Doreen Virtue has written this process out so clearly in her book, *How to Hear Your Angels.*[7] The following is a combination of her information and my own experience.

Develop your Intuition

There are four ways in which you can deepen your connection with your intuition.

1. **Clairsentience or** *clear-feeling*. This form of intuition comes from your feelings and physical sensations. When you begin to develop this sense, it is important to slow down and notice how you feel in certain situations.

You can probably remember a time when your *gut* told you not to enter into a relationship or a job and you did it anyway. Later you regretted it. Paying attention to these incidents allows you to have faith and learn to listen to your inner guidance. Listening to the inner guidance is a way of connecting directly with your Higher Self.

Start to become aware when you sense an angel around you or someone who has passed over. You may notice a familiar scent worn by a loved one, or smell fire or flowers when they are not present. You may feel your hair being stroked or feel as if you are being surrounded with a hug. You could sense someone sitting next to you when the being is not in physical form.[8]

It may be helpful to keep a journal of your senses and become more aware of the information you pick up. In fact, log in your journal any experiences you can remember regarding these four manners of connecting with your intuition.

2. **Claircognizance or *clear-knowing*.** This is when you find you simply know something but cannot explain why. This information may be coming from your Higher Self, or you may be tapping into the collective unconscious (Carl Jung's concept involving the universal repository of all religious, spiritual, and mythological symbols and experiences, as I explained earlier). The

difference between someone like me—a person who works as a clairvoyant—and other individuals is the fact that I listen to this voice. Don't do what we call *intellectual override*, in which you doubt the information you receive or think everybody knows the information. Practice listening to what you know.

Examples of this kind of awareness include meeting someone and already knowing details about them, or perhaps even having information regarding a current event about which you didn't read or hear.[9] Maybe you had an idea for a business plan or a book and didn't follow up on it, and someone else created the plan and became successful. Maybe you lost your keys and could close your eyes to see where they were. One instance that happens for me is that I usually know immediately 'who did it' when I watch detective shows.

In your journal, as you go through your day, note times when you have a hunch about something. Then notice when it comes true for you. This might be a feeling that someone will call or that a certain something will arrive in the mail. It could also be a sense that an appointment is going to be cancelled, or you may not want to schedule something that day because you have a feeling that something previously unexpected will happen. Also, watch when you doubt yourself, and note when you were right in spite of your doubt.

3. **Clairaudience or** *clear-hearing*. This is when you hear information. These voices can be from different sources. When you hear information, ask who is talking to you. Information from God is loud and to the point.[10] It is friendly, casual, and conveyed in modern language.[11] Archangels are also loud and to the point, but they are more formal and direct.[12] They often talk about getting on track with your goals and not being fearful or doubting yourself. Angels are also formal and direct.[13] Our deceased loved ones sound the way they did when they were physically alive.[14]

Our Higher Self sounds like our own voice and is supportive and loving. Our Ego comes across as abusive, discouraging, paranoid, and depressing. When I ask a question and am not sure if the response is coming from my Ego, I then go higher into the heavens and ask again. I can usually discern between my Higher Self and my Ego. Listen and start to distinguish your Higher Self from your Ego.

Become aware of the voices you hear. Just let it happen and don't analyze; instead, listen and make notes in your journal.

4. **Clairvoyance or** *clear-seeing*. With clairvoyance, you may see images and understand a meaning associated with these visions. Some come through dreams, and others can come with your eyes

closed or open. Be aware of your dreams and the images that come to you with your eyes closed. Record these images and other intuitive experiences in your journal, and begin to see a pattern of information from your Higher Self.

Another example of nurturing clairvoyance is seeing an incredible bird fly by and then being aware of what you were thinking right before it happened. This can be a message. Also, when you find coins or feathers on the ground, this could be a connection from your Higher Self, an angel, or someone who has passed over. Again, make notes in your journal regarding what you see.

According to Virtue, you can determine whether the information you are getting through clairsentience, claircognizance, clairaudience, and/or clairvoyance is true if it displays the following characteristics:[15]

1. Consistent—you get it more than once, or you get it over and over.

2. Motivating—you are guided to help others or improve a situation, not to get rich or famous.

3. Positive tone—the sense is uplifting and joyful. (False information is critical and negative.)

4. Clear origination—you get the information quickly and clearly. (False information comes after worry and is stressful.)

5. Familiarity – the guidance fits with who you are, as well as your skills and talents. It is something familiar to you.

Those whose representational systems are visual often also intuit through visual images. The images are often representational or symbolic, but they can be literal as well.

With a wide range of information available on the Internet and certain changes in mainstream television, my hope is that times have changed and children will feel accepted and learn to cultivate their intuitive abilities. I am often asked about how I developed my own psychic ability and whether or not I was psychic as a child. If you asked me the same question twenty years ago, I would not have understood my psychic ability the way I do today. When I was a child, I sensed that most of my important experiences took place in the nighttime and my dreamtime. I remember saying to people as a young child, "I only get through the day to get into the night where things really happen."

I didn't realize then what I do now; I complete most of my personal healing work with individuals and the planet at nighttime. Sometimes these are people I know and love, and other times I find myself energetically at a site where there has been a crisis, such as an earthquake or a hurricane. When I hear about the crisis the next day, I cry uncontrollably in sensing I had been there helping. The crying is like a clearing for me—not really painful, but releasing.

Though I didn't realize it was healing work as a child, I was very aware that my dreams were significant to me. Living in a violent home with an alcoholic father and a mother who was overwhelmed by emotional and physical pain, daily life held a lot of tension. On the other hand, my dreams were fun, creative, relaxing, and safe. I dreamed that my father, an auto mechanic in real life, was a sheriff similar to Andy Griffith of *Mayberry RFD*. I do want to add here that my father was violent toward my mom but not toward me. He loved me and was my main nurturer. Although I didn't understand it at the time, my father relied on me rather than my mother for his emotional needs, a phenomenon that is not uncommon and one that demonstrates a lack of boundaries.

As a child and young woman, I was very sensitive. I felt many different sensations, often in my gut. I knew something was wrong, but I couldn't figure out what the sensations meant. How wonderful it would have been if, when my tummy hurt (which was often), my mother or father would have known how to talk with me and help me figure out what I was feeling. My father always told me, "You are too emotional."

Today we are more aware of sensitives, which I will explain further below. We understand that those who access intuitive information naturally are gifted. When they are children, we can guide them and validate the information they receive. As a child, I knew when something was wrong. I could feel it in my body, but given my low self-esteem, I took this sign to mean something was wrong with me. After several traumatic experiences, I finally learned to trust my own inner guidance, but it took years. I now realize that many of the emotions I felt were not my own. As a sensitive, I was picking up on my father's anger and my mother's pain. This is a simplified version of the story, as I had an older and younger brother, and the home was extremely dysfunctional at times.

I have come to believe over the years that sensitives suffer from chronic pain and other illnesses—including alcoholism and drug addiction—more than others do.

Sensitives

In her book, *The Sensitive Person's Survival Guide*, Kyra Mesich describes the experience she had in taking on one of her client's feelings.[16] Mesich was not aware that this transference was taking place.

One evening, after working as a psychologist at a counseling center all day, Mesich was engaging in her usual after-work activities. She reported that after finishing the dishes, "Suddenly my mood changed. I was overtaken by a wash of sickening depression that seemed to come out of nowhere ... a dark abyss had opened, and I was promptly falling in. This dark depression came on so suddenly it took me aback."[17] The depression continued through the night, though Mesich did whatever she could to try and change it, including reading, listening to music, and engaging in light exercise; nothing worked. She ended up in tears. She kept thinking, "I am a failure. There is no hope for my future. I've screwed up my life. Things will never change."[18] She wrote in her journal and was confused by the feelings she had, because they didn't make any sense. They didn't reflect her life.

The next day at work, she found that her secretary had scheduled an appointment during her lunch hour with a client who had urgently requested that she see him. When Mesich met with this client, Dan, he shared a poem with her that he had written showing extreme sadness and depression. He said he had experienced "an especially painful depressive episode" the previous night.[19] Rebuffed by a woman, the dialogue trailing through his mind over and over was, "I am a complete failure. I've screwed up my life beyond repair. I have no hope for my future. Things will never change."[20] When Mesich asked him what prompted him to write the poem, he responded, "I was listening to my new Indigo Girls CD. There is a song on there that is so sad. I felt like it could have been the story of me. It inspired me to write my own words of my own pain. So late into the night I listened to that song and worked that poem."[21] Mesich described her feelings at the time:

> I hoped Dan didn't notice my mouth fall open in shock. I felt like a ton of bricks had just been dropped on top of me. I was baffled and dismayed. Dan had just described in perfect detail, every single facet of the depression I felt last night. It was uncanny. The intense quality of the emotional pain, the exact thoughts, the precise time the depression began, and now I found out that we had been listening to the same CD. The song that drove into me like a knife was the very song that inspired Dan to write his poem.[22]

This awareness was extremely distressing to Mesich, and she struggled with the fact that she was experiencing her client's feelings. She didn't feel Dan's feelings again in the same way but did experience many of her clients' feelings in the next several weeks. In fact, the very next week, Mesich had a panic attack at the same time her female client had one while was driving over a bridge.[23] She was concerned about the experience she was having. It wrought havoc on her life, and she and her supportive husband had many conversations about the phenomenon and what she could do. Researching the literature, she could not find any references to anything that was exactly like her experience.

Her emotions were volatile and she was frightened. In medical terms, she was experiencing what could be described as psychosis.[24]

A short while later, her husband was offered a position in another state, and they moved. Happy to leave her current situation, she decided to step away from the counseling field for a time and began working in an art gallery. During this time, she continued to do research and found a name for what had been occurring—*empathic ability*.[25] She also found that it was quite common and actually called "the most common psychic ability."[26]

After her move, Mesich realized she still picked up on the feelings of other people, or what I refer to as "matching" another's energy or emotions. She continued to research and found that the psychological community was beginning to understand the set of character traits that make up the sensitive person's experience.[27] The reason I am including this information is that I believe all physical pain has an emotional or spiritual basis, or both. Many of us who suffer from chronic pain have taken on the pain of others. Below is a list of attributes Mesich ascribes to emotionally sensitive people:

- Emotionally sensitive people feel emotions often and deeply. They feel as if they "wear their emotions on their sleeves."

- They are keenly aware of the emotions of people around them.

- Sensitive people are easily hurt or upset. An insult or unkind remark will affect them deeply.

- In a similar vein, sensitive people strive to avoid conflict. They dread arguments and other types of confrontations because the negativity affects them so much.

- Sensitive people are not able to shake off emotions easily. Once they are saddened or upset by something, they cannot just switch gears and forget it.

- Sensitive people are greatly affected by the emotions they witness. They feel deeply for the suffering of others. Many sensitive people avoid sad movies or watching the news because they cannot bear the weighty emotions that would drive to their core and stick with them afterwards.

- Sensitive people are prone to suffer from recurrent depression, anxiety, or other psychological disorders.

- On the positive side, sensitive people are also keenly aware of and affected by beauty in art, music, and nature. They are the world's greatest artists and art appreciators.

- Sensitive people are prone to stimulus overload. That is, they can't stand large crowds, loud noise, or hectic environments. They feel overwhelmed and depleted by too much stimulation.

- Sensitive people are born that way. They were sensitive children. There are a couple of different responses kids have to their sensitivity. One type of sensitive child is the stereotypical kid who gets picked on by bullies, and is a well-behaved, good student because he or she cannot stand the thought of getting into trouble. The other type of sensitive child more often experiences the stimulus overload mentioned in the previous paragraph. These children are thus over-stimulated and have difficulty focusing, which causes them problems in school.[28]

Your pain may or may not relate to sensitivity, so it is important to assess yourself to determine which is true for you. The tools in this book are all helpful tools for sensitive people. If you find you are sensitive, it is helpful to research and learn more about this and to find people in your local community who are sensitive as well. You will most likely find them in meditation groups, dream groups, and alternative medicine circles. It is often the sensitive people who are in the alternative medicine fields.

Similar to Dr. Mesich's fear that her colleagues would think her psychotic, as my own intuitive abilities began to develop, I was resistant to sharing my experiences with my coworkers. Over the years I have been developing the idea of a book I would write: *If I Weren't So Spiritual, I Think I'd Be Crazy!*

As it happened, I began to attend a church called the Church of Divine Man in Spokane, Washington, and there began my study of metaphysics. I was delighted to find people like myself there, and I took a class on healing and another on meditation. Though I didn't continue attending, I did receive a few psychic readings. After doing so one day, I was on my stair-stepper when I saw all of my chakras on a screen before me, and I could read them! It was instantaneous, and that was the beginning of reading myself.

Later that year, I offered to perform healings with a friend that had volunteered to do acupuncture at a retreat comprised of people who were HIV positive or had AIDS. The people at the retreat were extremely responsive. I performed many healings, moving energy around and through chakras, and my wrist hurt for days afterward. The really exciting part was that—because I had done so many healings in such a short time—I automatically began to read people's chakras, offering them information on where blocks existed and what they needed to do to heal. Their openness to my information and healing work validated my new ability so strongly that I was motivated to continue practicing and learning.

Not long after this, a friend and I decided to practice performing readings on each other. At first I hated doing these readings. The energy coming through my body was so intense that it felt uncomfortable. I also noticed that my friend and I read differently, although we used the same process. She was a nurse, and when she read me, she saw the physical characteristics of my body—both inside and out. In my reading of her, as a mental health counselor, I read the emotional issues and energy connected to behaviors that were stuck in her chakras.

Many people look for medical intuitive readings. With study, I learned that all physical issues relate to emotional issues and, at the core, to the belief beneath those emotions. With this knowledge, I began adding psychic readings to my private practice. As I practiced over time, I started getting other information. For example, when conducting a reading on a client, one of the client's family members would show up energetically. Often the family member would show up angry, feeling protective of the loved one sitting in front of me. Usually, once the family member connected with my energy, that person asked me for a healing as well.

At other times in reading a client, I would just naturally tone, making sounds from deep within myself (you will read my original story about healing through toning in Week Ten). This sound would quickly move any foreign energy in the energy field of the client, and most often any pain or unusual sensation would disappear. When doing the toning, I would often sense a connection with ancient shamans, and they would use my voice for healing. It appeared they were channeling through me.

I feel a strong connection to shamanism, although I have not studied much about it. There is something that stirs deep within when I begin to tone. Maybe that is because shamanism deals with the underworld or the unconscious part of us that many never bring into consciousness. You may get a better understanding of this if you experience a drumming circle or just listen to some shamanistic drumming music. It is such a sensational response that language becomes obsolete.

Eventually I became very comfortable with my readings. Later I realized that my head injury experience also contributed to my psychic ability. When I was fourteen years old, I accepted a ride while waiting at a bus stop. The driver was a younger man who drove a light blue Ford or Chevy truck. I was what was referred to as a "Jesus Freak" at the time. We had newspapers that we passed out to all, called "The Truth." I was on my way downtown to witness for Jesus. I remember thinking as I entered the truck, "Jesus will take care of me."

The next conscious awareness I had was of looking up at the lights at Holy Family Hospital and seeing my mom and dad looking back at me. I had a contusion, which is a serious head injury. I was told that the priest had administered the last rites as I had been unconscious for two weeks and was not expected to live. The doctors told my parents that if I were to live, it was not at all certain I would recover.

During this coma, I had a near-death experience and saw myself going through the tunnel. I felt sensations all around me, like I was floating in a swirl of energy. There was also a light greyness around me, and I could see the light ahead. As I came closer to the light, I witnessed a few angel-like beings. A male voice told me I was not ready to leave and that I had to go back and finish my life.

As I recovered, I was extremely angry. It was difficult learning to think and use my limbs again. My brain was injured, I experienced petit mal epilepsy seizures, and I had a difficult time remembering anything. I realized later that because I could not function in a normal way, I had to rely on my intuitive senses to survive. This method of compensation increased my intuitive ability.

Once I miraculously recovered, I became curious about what had happened to put me in the hospital. The police informed me that the man who had picked me up was not taking me downtown, but was instead taking me behind Albi Stadium, a secluded place far from downtown. I apparently exited the car somehow, but we didn't know whether I had jumped out or he pushed me out.

Years later, I found the name of a counselor who was also a hypnotherapist, and I made an appointment. In the first appointment, he began the induction process. I didn't really know anything about hypnotherapy and had not been prepared. I felt extremely vulnerable and was not able to focus or enter trance, which left me embarrassed and scared. Without expressing any of this, I just thanked him and left, feeling like a failure and very vulnerable. I understand now that it was necessary for me to have developed trust with this man prior to going into trance, especially given that my abductor had been a male of about the same age as the hypnotherapist.

Since then, I have had an incredibly positive hypnotherapy session with Dr. Gil Milner, who took me back to that experience, and I was able to relive the experience in great detail and heal the trauma. As it turned out, my abductor was turning a corner quickly as I had a hold on the door handle, readying myself to exit. I flew out of the truck and landed on my head. It is a blessing that I have recovered as well as I have.

So, in summary, my psychic ability was present in childhood, just as it is for most children. The ability increased due to my head injury when brain damage forced me to use other senses. It developed more as I took classes to learn the process of psychic reading. And—as with everything else in life—my psychic capabilities expanded with practice, practice, and more practice. Other ways to cultivate your own intuitive abilities include prayer and meditation, which I will address in Week Eight.

Self-Talk

In the late 1990s, I was the clinical director of a chemical dependency agency in Spokane, Washington. The team of counselors and I went through training for certification in reality therapy, a concept developed by Dr. William Glasser. Incorporating this information with data gleaned from

Glasser's book, *Choice Theory*, we developed a cognitive behavioral treatment program.[29] This was an alternative to the 12-step programs that were the current mainstay of treatment in the field.

At that time, I was married to a man who also worked at the agency. We had completed the certification together and both tended to be what I refer to as "heady." Our conversations were often intellectual and creative. What I found was the pattern of getting home from work, having a nice dinner cooked by my husband, and resting. When it was time to sleep, my mind would race and I'd ruminate for hours. Continually reliving the day, reworking conversations, and second-guessing my choices in words or works wasn't conducive to sleep! I was very aware of my self-talk. Although it was not always negative, it was all-encompassing. Choosing to just live with it, I accepted my self-talk as a necessary evil in running a treatment program.

I have since learned to challenge the negative self-talk and quiet my mind. This was done through a deliberate and challenging process using hypnotherapy, which we covered in Week Four, as well as meditation, which is covered in Week Eight. While you can feel free to take a peek ahead or revisit sections as necessary for a better understanding of the two, we will now explore how you can stop the chatter in your head and replace it with loving, supportive thoughts.

Let's start by talking about the danger and drawback in the whole New Age concept of "creating with our beliefs." Given the premise that we create and manifest with our beliefs, the natural next step is to believe we create our illness. At some level this is true, but I remember information I learned in attending a workshop called Medical Intuition Training in April 2004, taught by Caroline

Myss and Norm Shealy.[30] Myss said that most of us are not able to manifest healing or create illness instantaneously, because in order to do so, we need to have our attention in present time. Most of us hold our attention in the past or future. Works on energy medicine often explain that illness is created in our etheric field—our subtle energy body that is *around* our body—years before it manifests *within* our body. With this premise, I would like to look at how we can change our thoughts and heal our bodies.

In his 1990 book, *Quantum Healing: Exploring the Frontiers of Mind/Body Medicine*, Deepak Chopra said he "would argue that our inner space is a rich field of silent intelligence, and that it exerts a powerful influence on us."[31] Although we have a constant stream of consciousness, Chopra focuses on the healing aspect of your inner self as this silent intelligence, which he explains to be the silent gap between your thoughts.[32] He elaborates: "The universe was created once, but we re-create ourselves with every thought."[33] When discussing whether it is the head or heart that determines our interpretation of situations, he explains, "Something deeper, in the realm of silence, creates our view of reality."[34] It is the constant chatter in your mind that keeps you from this inner intelligence, which is the part of you that is all-intelligent; it is this constant chatter that keeps you from the self-healing part of your being.

Chopra notes, "It is possible to spend a lifetime listening to the inventory of the mind without ever dipping into its source."[35] We must learn to access the gap between each thought, which is the place in which the intelligence lies. Chopra suggests that just before falling asleep, the mind gradually leaves the waking state. It withdraws the senses, shuts out the waking world, and a brief gap opens at the junction point before the mind actually falls asleep. This gap is identical to the one that flashes by between each thought. It is a like a little window into the field that is beyond either wakefulness or sleep.[36]

I also described this light trance "twilight state" in the week on hypnotherapy. It is a good time to give yourself suggestions, as well as to go inward to your own inner silence.

Chopra writes, "Subjective reality and objective reality are tightly bound together."[37] He appears to agree with Glasser when he opines, "When the mind shifts, the body cannot help but follow. Objective reality looks obviously more fixed than our subjective moods, fleeting desires, and swings of emotion. Yet perhaps it is not; it is more like a violin string that can hold one pitch but also change pitch as your finger slides along it."[38]

Chopra adds, "The pitch on the string stands for your level of consciousness."[39] He explains that our pitch does not change easily. Instead, it is similar to how we look at the world. We may be looking at the world through green glasses, whereas someone else may have orange glasses. Let's say the green glasses have a feeling similar to anger. When an angry person walks into the room, even though nothing is said, the whole room changes, and you can feel it. What you are feeling is this person's pitch. And you cannot change your pitch by simply thinking it so. As Chopra puts it:

> Everything you think and do is determined by this point— you cannot think yourself to a higher or lower level of consciousness. This helps explain why meditation is not simply another kind of thinking or introspection, a mistake Westerners tend to make. It is actually a way to slide to a new pitch. The process of transcending, or "going beyond," detaches the mind from its fixed level and allows it to exist, if only for a moment,

without any level at all. It simply experiences silence, devoid of thoughts, emotions, desires, wishes, fear, or anything at all. Afterward, when the mind returns to its usual pitch (level of consciousness), it has acquired a little freedom to move.[40]

For the purpose of this book, which is to understand that all healing is self-healing, it is important to fully share Chopra's view. He explains:

From a medical standpoint, a disease may represent a place on the violin string that is out of tune. Yet, for some reason, the mind-body system cannot find a way to let go, to slide to a healthier pitch. If that is so, then meditation may be a powerful therapeutic tool, allowing the body to get unstuck from the disease. Meditation researchers caught on to this potential in the late 1960s when they discovered that college-age meditators who used alcohol, cigarettes, and recreational drugs spontaneously quit their habit within a few months of beginning to meditate. We can call this getting unstuck from an old level of consciousness that needed the drug; in terms of neuropeptides, it may be the meditation freed up certain receptor sites by offering molecules that were more satisfying than alcohol, nicotine, or marijuana.[41]

We all know that children from an early age mimic their parents. My family has a cute picture of my now deceased older brother Cary sitting on a bench at about age two with a cigarette in his mouth, trying to light it. This was cute, because it was decades before the dangers of cigarettes entered mainstream thought. Looking back now, my brother died of alcoholism at age thirty-seven, my mother of cancer directly related to cigarettes at age fifty-six, and my father of cancer directly related to cigarettes at age seventy. In discussing studies of chimps mimicking their parents, Bruce Lipton concludes, "In humans as well, the fundamental behaviors, beliefs, and attitudes we observe in our parents become 'hard-wired' as synaptic pathways in our subconscious minds."[42] He continues by explaining the following:

> [C]ells, which can teach us so much about ourselves ... are intelligent. But remember, when cells band together in creating multicellular communities, they follow the "collective voice" of the organism, even if that voice dictates self-destructive behavior. Our physiology and behavior patterns conform to the "truths" of the central voice, be they constructive or destructive beliefs.[43]

An internationally recognized leader in bridging science and spirit, Dr. Bruce Lipton attributes this unwavering "central voice" adherence to the power of the subconscious, which is "an emotionless database of stored programs whose function is strictly concerned with reading environmental signals and engaging in hard-wired behavioral programs."[44] An example of this automatic playback from the subconscious shows up often in the form of your buttons getting pushed!

Lipton refers to our subconscious mind as our autopilot and the conscious mind as the manual control.[45] The subconscious mind processes about 20,000,000 environmental stimuli a second, whereas the conscious mind processes about 40 environmental stimuli in the same second. We have free will with the conscious mind; however, whenever we are not conscious, not aware, or not paying attention, the subconscious mind takes over. Although this can be good when you are driving a car, it is not as advantageous in many other instances, including self-reflection. Your subconscious mind is full of behaviors and beliefs that come from others, such as your parents, family, teachers, ministers, television, and anyone who has influenced your learning. Many of us didn't experience the loving homes we would have liked to have had and thus have deep thoughts in our subconscious of being less than, undeserving, or unworthy.

Although the ideal is to have had the perfect parenting and introduction into the world, it often does not happen this way. In my private counseling practice, I have worked with hundreds of clients in helping them to re-parent themselves. Today, in addition to using re-parenting, I work more directly through the subconscious and use hypnosis to install suggestions that override the previous ones. You can do this with the tools you learned in the third week. Also, eye movement desensitization and reprocessing (EMDR) is an effective treatment, especially for trauma. I will talk more about this technique in the sixth week.

Healing and Healers

When I say that all healing is self-healing, I wonder how you respond. Think for a moment … when was the first time you thought of healing or of healers? Given your experience, there can be several different connotations for these words and this concept. I know that between my family members' table talk of maladies and my first major experience with doctors coming from a hospital when I nearly died, I have rarely chosen to go to doctors since, instead preferring to do whatever I can to find solutions that do not involve the white coats. And yes, while this represents a part of myself that I yet have to resolve, it has also opened my mind to other solutions regarding health problems.

My mother was often ill when I was a child, and she frequently went to the doctor. I don't remember there being any talk of healing in or around my home, despite all that talk of doctors. I went to a Nazarene Church when I was young, and other than when I snuck out of the house to go to the Baptist Church around the corner (must have been the music), I was not aware of spiritual healing until I converted to Catholicism in 1979. There is a part of me that envies those who grew up in a home where the women naturally laid hands on those who were suffering. Today, in having become a Reiki Master in 1991 and teaching Reiki since, I definitely see myself as a healer. I believe we are all healers.

In my own healing practice, I have learned to focus inward and center myself. By this I mean that I quiet myself in my heart and ground myself. I then bring my attention and consciousness up into the heavens and ask the Divine to allow a healing for the person with whom I am working. If I am using Reiki with the client, I use the Reiki symbols that are used by Reiki practitioners. Spiritual healers and prayer healers usually center themselves and connect with energy beyond themselves. This could mean connecting with God, Goddess, healing Guides, Jesus, the Universe, or their Higher Power. When I work with clients, I generally ask them, "To Whom do you pray?" I then use my own healing guides and theirs as well.

When entering into a prayerful healing session, most studies show that the best results come from praying with a positive—but not determined—expectation. You ask for healing in a state of receptive, loving, peace and quiet. You may feel energy coming from the top of your head down into your body, but the results of the healing are left up to the being or entity to whom you pray.

When I talk about self-healing, I think about life as if it were a movie. The stopped frame of your life right now may show you with an illness, but if you fast-forward, you might see the illness was a catalyst that brought about greater happiness and health at the end of the reel. This has been shown to be the case time and again. Many of us are aware of those who've suffered from heart attacks and have changed their lifestyle as a result. Have you heard of such an example in which someone experienced a life-threatening disease or event and is now happier than ever before? Perhaps they are more grateful and accepting of life. Maybe they work less and enjoy their family and life passions more. Of course you've heard or witnessed stories of extreme illness acting as a catalyst for positive change. No matter the example or potential repercussions, it's clear that we cannot know for sure what great gift an illness may be giving. The healing can come at many levels. It may be evidenced on the spiritual, mental, emotional, or physical level. All of this is self-healing.

In his 2001 book, *Vibrational Medicine*, Richard Gerber writes about Dan Winter's discovery of a resonant energy connection between the loving energy of healers and our planet's magnetic energy field.[46] This is a discovery that reveals many possibilities. During sessions between healers and patients, studies showed brain wave activity at about 7.8 Hz (cycles per second). This is the "alpha-theta interface and the so-called Schumann resonance of the Earth's magnetic field," which is the nurturing Mother Earth energy that feeds living cells and heals the environment.[47] Gerber proposes that the 7.8 frequency allows for a resonance-frequency window through which energy cascades like a magnetic waterfall of the planetary field, and healers become a conduit of the energy flow.

He also believes that "healers not only emit subtle magnetic fields that are coherent, but these healing fields produce coherence in other energy fields around them, both locally and nonlocally."[48] What he means by this is that healers increase both local and distance coherence in Earth's magnetic field itself. The healing from many healers becomes exponential. Therefore, healers are not merely a conduit of healing; in the healing, they also send forth this magnetic energy back to the Earth. Healers and meditators who focus this loving energy to the planet may shift the planet to a higher vibration. I am familiar with this concept, and my initial "awakening" in 1991 was quickly followed by connecting with others all over the planet, dressing in white, focusing in our hearts, and walking in formations. Our intention was to bring in light and love from the planet and to awaken it to a higher vibration in this 11:11 ceremony (see **http://www.nvisible .com**).[49]

Gerber surmises that the difficulty in healing the planet is the need to heal ourselves first. This is my belief as well, so what I find most important in all that I do is the act of raising my own vibration in order to contribute to raising our planet's vibration. I would also like to teach you to do the same. On my 1990 CD, *Chakra Clearing*, I take you through a process of grounding and self-healing that focuses on the chakras.[50] With the material on this CD, I help you to raise the vibration of your own frequency.

Gerber further explains the following, with respect to healing:

> Laying-on-of-hands healing has been practiced throughout the world for thousands of years. In the late 1700s, Franz Mesmer theorized that subtle life energy of a magnetic nature was exchanged between healer and patient during laying-on-of-

hands. Mesmer also discovered that water could effectively store this subtle force for transfer to sick patients in need of healing.[51]

In teaching Reiki healing for many years, I have told my students that we all have the ability to heal. Many clients experienced their own ability to feel energy and heal themselves as well as others in this process.

An illustration of this principle involved a client of mine with cancer who was in the hospital preparing for surgery. I asked my students to meet me there and use Reiki to help calm her and assist in the healing process. When the doctors located a blood clot and could not operate, I invited my students, as well as the client's mother and sister, to assist me in laying hands on the client. After talking with the nurse in charge, I understood the clot needed to dissolve before they could operate. We all imaged this as we did the healing. A period of a half hour or so went by, and when I felt an immediate sense that the healing was complete, I asked the nurse to check again. They did, and the clot was gone. The client was subsequently able to receive the needed surgery, the mother and sister of the patient were able to be helpful, and my students' confidence in their healing ability increased. It was a glorious day!

We are all connected to the Source, and we all have the ability to channel this love. Here are some exercises to practice so that you can define your beliefs and connect with the God of your heart, as well as get in touch with your own healing abilities.

Tools and Exercises

Try a few of these exercises, and just be aware of your response to them. You will find what works best for you.

1. Take some time to think about your beliefs. Talk with your friends and family about them, and journal as well. You can do so in the following format:

   A. Write about your attitudes, viewpoints, ideas, thoughts, values, and perceptions that are absolute. They are unchangeable.

   B. Write down attitudes, viewpoints, ideas, thoughts, values, and perceptions that you are unsure about. They may be changeable.

   C. Write about attitudes, viewpoints, ideas, thoughts, values, and perceptions that you would be terrified to change.

   D. What are your attitudes, viewpoints, ideas, thoughts, values, and perceptions that keep you ill?

   E. What attitudes, viewpoints, ideas, thoughts, values, and perceptions may allow you to heal?

2. Starting with childhood and continuing to adulthood, list some memories of being intuitive. Whom did you tell about your experience, and how did they respond? Begin to journal your intuitive experiences, and look them over at the

end of each week. The more you practice and notice this ability, the greater it becomes.

3. Go to the NLP Word List in appendix 2, and circle the words you find yourself using often. Are you more visual, auditory, kinesthetic, olfactory, or gustatory? Start to listen to your friends and family to see what words they use the most. This is a great exercise to figure out the best gifts for your loved ones. For example, if you have a friend who is visual, you may want to get them something they can read or see, such as a map or a book. A loved one who is kinesthetic would love something with texture, such as a fuzzy or silky gift. Auditory friends would like music or audio books more than a visual friend. Someone who has a great olfactory sense would like something that has a great scent, or maybe even a weekend in the woods. And the friend whose primary sense is gustatory would enjoy food and drink!

4. Reread the section on developing your intuition and note in your journal your main way of obtaining intuitive information. We are much more open to listening to our inner self when we are young. (No wonder author J.K. Rowling had Harry Potter begin his experiences with the world of magic at age ten!) Write about what you were doing and feeling in life when you were ten to twelve years old. Use the journal process of free writing you learned in the first week to remember some of your experiences as a child.

5. Practice hands-on healing on yourself. When you are stressed or in pain, gently lay your hands on your body and breathe. You may want to focus on your heart, allowing yourself to feel love there, and notice what happens in your hands and to the part of your body you are healing.

6. Having read about the subconscious and conscious minds, write out some beliefs you would like to change. Use the self-hypnosis tools you learned in the third week to change these beliefs. You can do this by intention. Write down the belief, and allow your subconscious mind to grant your intention.

Week Six: Stress Comes in Many Forms

Many people think about stress as being specific to negative happenings in their lives, but stress actually occurs from both negative and positive situations. In fact, your energy system picks up a great amount of stress without you even being aware. What's wonderful, however, is that your body is amazing at moving back into balance.

You may remember a time when something happened suddenly and unexpectedly, and you immediately went into a heightened state of awareness. Your body is set up with a protective mechanism toward "fight" or "flight." This reaction creates an outpouring of adrenaline and other hormones into your blood stream, which produces a number of protective changes in your body. This flood provides you with the energy and strength to either fight or flee from the situation. Here, your heart rate increases, allowing more blood flow to your muscles, brain, and heart. Your breathing also increases to a faster pace in order to take in more oxygen, and your muscles tense in preparation for action. You become mentally alert, and your senses become more aware so that you can assess the situation and act quickly. In addition to this, your blood sugar, fats, and cholesterol increase for extra energy. There is a rise in your platelets and blood clotting ability, which prevents hemorrhaging in case of injury.

Most of the time though, you don't have this fight-or-flight response. Instead, there is a steady stream of stressors that increase and decrease as the day goes on. You become accustomed to the stress and then see it as normal, and all the while it is taking a toll on your body. You may find you compare yourself to others and then think that you don't have it so bad, or that your stress is worse than others, which creates more stress.

This makes me remember the frog metaphor. One frog is put in a pot of boiling water and quickly jumps out. Another is put in a pot of cold water and the temperature is heated slowly. The latter frog adjusts to the temperature and dies. When you have a traumatic stress, you tend to react and move away from the situation, but if the stress is gradual— even if it is traumatic—you may stay. This is the case with people who are in abusive relationships. Little by little, they develop what is termed *learned helplessness* and have a difficult time leaving the relationship. This could be the case with illness as well. Some people take action and develop the strengths they can to excel in their lives, and others allow the pain to overtake them.

If this makes you wonder about your own stress level, there are several stress tests you can take. The one I use is the Holmes and Rahe Stress Scale. It is a standard test developed initially in 1967 by two psychiatrists, Thomas Holmes and Richard Rahe.[1] This test was published as the Social Readjustment Rating Scale (SRRS). Using Life Change Units (LCU), they were able to correlate the relationship between stress and illness in participants. In 1970, Rahe implemented another test, which assessed the reliability of the stress scale as a predictor of illness.[2] Take a moment to evaluate your stress level with this test (see Figure 4).

Life event	Life change units
Death of a spouse	100
Divorce	73
Marital separation	65
Imprisonment	63
Death of a close family member	63
Personal injury or illness	53
Marriage	50
Dismissal from work	47
Marital reconciliation	45
Retirement	45
Change in health of family member	44
Pregnancy	40
Sexual difficulties	39
Gain a new family member	39
Business readjustment	39
Change in financial state	38
Death of a close friend	37
Change to different line of work	36
Change in frequency of arguments	35
Major mortgage	32
Foreclosure of mortgage or loan	30
Change in responsibilities at work	29
Child leaving home	29
Trouble with in-laws	29
Outstanding personal achievement	28
Spouse starts or stops work	26
Begin or end school	26
Change in living conditions	25
Revision of personal habits	24

Life event	Life change units
Trouble with boss	23
Change in working hours or conditions	20
Change in residence	20
Change in schools	20
Change in recreation	19
Change in church activities	19
Change in social activities	18
Minor mortgage or loan	17
Change in sleeping habits	16
Change in number of family reunions	15
Change in eating habits	15
Vacation	13
Christmas	12
Minor violation of law	11

Figure 4 The Social Readjustment Rating Scale

Score of 300+: At risk of illness.
Score of 150–299: Risk of illness is moderate
(reduced by 30% from the above risk).
Score 150–: Only have a slight risk of illness.

Having taken the test, you may be surprised by the results. If you find you do not have many of the stressors listed but still struggle with stress, understand that although we share a human experience, we all experience life differently. You may have noticed this when you read about sensitives in Week Five. You may also find that you have many more stressors in your life than you would have thought. If this is the case, don't be alarmed. There is a solution, and we will spend the bulk of this section covering it. Each item is italicized and then listed again for you to be able to easily scan in the future as a refresher.

In addition to understanding what stresses you, I've created a list of stress symptoms you may note experiencing. All of the symptoms I list here can be overwhelming and exhausting. Physical symptoms you may notice when stressed include increased heart rate, pounding heart, elevated blood pressure, sweaty palms, headache, diarrhea, constipation, urinary hesitancy, trembling, twitching, stuttering, nausea, vomiting, sleep disturbances, fatigue, shallow breathing, dry mouth, cold hands, itching, being easily startled, chronic pain, susceptibility to illness, and tightness in the chest, neck, jaw, and back muscles.

Emotional signs and symptoms of stress include irritability, angry outbursts, hostility, depression, jealousy, restlessness, withdrawal, anxiousness, diminished initiative, hyper-vigilance, feeling that things are not real, lack of interest in things you used to enjoy, crying outbursts, being critical of others, self-deprecation, nightmares, impatience, lack of hope, narrowed focus, obsessive rumination, lack of self-esteem, insomnia, and either overeating or loss of appetite.

In addition to taking the Holmes and Rahe Stress test mentioned earlier, before you make changes, figure out on a scale from 1–10 how stressed you feel in your life. Do this with 1 being little or no stress, 5 being a medium level of stress (or being stressed about half the time during the week), and 10 being a high level of stress (or being stressed daily). Make a note of your stress score in your journal so you can test yourself again after using some of the tools outlined for you.

Now that you know your stress level and what your stressors are, what can you do? The first suggestion I have is to learn to be in *present time*; this means to learn to focus in the present moment. When your mind wanders to the future or the past, bring it back. One way to do this is to breathe and focus on the sensations in your body for a moment, which is quite effective in bringing you back to present time. You will soon learn that your body feels safe and comfortable when you are in present time. When you are not, you may immediately feel scattered. It does take practice, but it feels great.

It is also often helpful to *compartmentalize* your life. What I mean by this is to focus on one thing at a time. A friend of mine calls this "mouse medicine." Only focus on the one activity you are doing until you are finished, and then move to the next. It used to be said that multi-tasking was a good idea, but more recently I have heard and begun to believe myself that staying focused on one task at a time is better. Completing tasks this way can be less stressful. And while you are handling that moment's one task, keep your mind consciously focused there.

Often you can lessen your stress by having *realistic deadlines and goals*. When I was getting ready to complete the manuscript for this book and send it to the editor, I had set a deadline for myself that was unrealistic. My response to this was to panic, and my body just shut down; I couldn't focus, couldn't think, and found my hand reaching out for a sugary treat to numb myself. I quickly figured this was not the best option and subsequently called the editor to change the deadline. Once I changed the deadline, I was happy to continue writing and re-writing. Not only that, but I also felt so supported by my editor that it actually helped motivate me, and I realized I don't have to do everything alone.

You can also avoid procrastination by *breaking projects down into manageable pieces.* Put these smaller pieces and goals toward the greater whole either on your calendar or a note attached to your mirror, refrigerator, or office white board. I also really like the idea of having an accountability partner. If you have a large project, break the project into segments and share with a friend or coworker who also has a project they can share with you. Have a predetermined time each week to hold each other accountable.

Few people are really balanced, although they often work toward it. You may either under-function or over-function. If you over-function, think about what is realistic for you. It is important to *know your limits* and to prioritize. This is especially important if your pain is changing your ability to function. There is always someone else who can do more. Allow yourself to honor your own self, and don't push too hard. Write out what is important and *prioritize.* Many people spend hours doing what is not important in the peak hours of the day. Think about what you have done in the last couple days. How much of it was not important or enjoyable?

Another way to reduce your stress is to *eat healthy* and *avoid sugary snacks.* Sugar and caffeine both provide quick energy followed by a lull in energy. They also seem to set up a pattern of needing more to get going and then feeling even more lethargic. Caffeine can certainly contribute to your anxiety and stress levels. The more you can reduce the amount of sugar and caffeine you intake, the less stressed you will feel. You may find that *decreasing or alleviating caffeine altogether* will help you significantly. Be aware that chocolate and some pain relievers contain caffeine as well. Given that coffee is addictive, I suggest moving to green tea for your health and allowing yourself an occasional coffee treat. If you do drink coffee, limit it to before noon. Many people I have talked to say they can drink coffee all day long and still sleep, but I wonder what the quality of that sleep is, in addition to their stress and anxiety levels. You can refer back to Week Three for more information on diet and eating healthy.

Also discussed in Week Three was exercise. *Move your body to release stress.* This is one of the most effective tools. Even if you have limited mobility, you can stretch to release tension. From walking and gentle yoga to aerobic exercise, you will receive the benefit of stress release. It would be remiss of me not to remind you that over-exercise can also stress your body. If you are stressed due to an emotional issue and not dealing with the underlying problem, exercising in excess can be a poor response. It is important to allow yourself to feel the feelings and deal with the underlying issue. You will find more about this process in Week Seven.

Sometimes it is really important to simply notice what is going on. Slowing down and taking a moment to just close your eyes and check in with your body is important. Notice what you are feeling. This will help you become more conscious of yourself. It will also help your body to feel safe. Too often, people numb themselves and don't want to be present in the body, but allowing yourself to be in the body is when and where the healing happens.

Another note on the list of ways to release stress is the need to *get enough sleep*. It is recommended that you experience at least 7–8 hours of sleep each night. If you do this most nights, it will help lessen your stress.

That being said, many people have a difficult time sleeping. If you are one of them, I suggest that you allow your body to begin to rest early in the evening. You can participate in activities that are restful, while eliminating stressful situations like watching action packed movies or playing intense computer games. It is also best to do your computer work earlier in the day. Avoiding food late in the day or being sure to eat smaller meals late in the day will also help you sleep easier. Food takes a long time to digest, and it is best done when you are awake. For myself, I find a green smoothie for dinner is the best way to sleep restfully. You can experiment for yourself.

While flying back from Japan a couple of years ago, I found myself stalled in airports and waiting long periods of time between flights. Feeling very stressed, my body was so tense that I ached. When I returned back to the United States, I was asked for whatever reason to go back through security for an extra search. In choosing not to go through the x-ray machine, I was given a hand search. When the woman ran her hands down my back, I was surprised to feel the energy just release from my body, and I realized *the importance of touch* when stressed. If you don't have an intimate relationship where you are touched often, and you don't have children or grandchildren to cuddle with, I strongly encourage you to allow yourself the healing experience of massage at least monthly, and preferably weekly.

You may have also become in the habit of self-medicating pain with alcohol. To lessen your stress though, you must *decrease or alleviate alcohol altogether.* Whether it is emotional pain, physical pain, or both, the alcohol only masks it. The underlying issue remains. When you can easily cover pain for a time with alcohol, you lose motivation to work on healing, and you eventually may lose motivation for most everything. There is also the risk of creating a dependency on the alcohol. In developing a tolerance, it will take more alcohol to numb the pain. Eventually, your primary issue may no longer be the pain, but instead consist of situations that arise from the addiction to alcohol. All of this contributes to your stress level, and you end up in a vicious cycle.

Speaking of addictions, smoking is another stress inducer. *Become a non-smoker*, and you will increase your health in many areas. Nicotine speeds up your heart, increases your blood pressure, and decreases the oxygen your body needs. Most people are aware of the many other reasons not to smoke, so I won't delve deeper here, but I do offer a free smoking cessation program that you can find on my website. I created this program in honor of my parents who died of cancer as a direct result of smoking. We have no family history of cancer otherwise, for which I am grateful!

You are learning several tools to *reduce stress through relaxation* in this book. They include self-hypnosis, breathing, and meditation. All of these have proven results, and you can do each easily. I find that grounding yourself through a visualization process and living in present time help as well. You can find some grounding and centering videos at **http://www.youtube.com/energymedicinedna**.

Sharing with your friends is extremely helpful when you are stressed about a situation. The caution here is to make sure you share in a way that you feel more relaxed afterward. If you have a tendency to share your concerns with someone who feeds into them, or if you tend to share the same concerns over and over again, this can create stress. Learning to let go and move on in your life can be the next step. The Serenity Prayer is great for this.

God, grant me the serenity to accept
the things I cannot change,

12 Weeks to Self-Healing

Courage to change the things I can,
And wisdom to know the difference.

Journaling is one of the best tools for stress. The process for journaling is in the beginning of this book. In addition to connecting to your inner self or Higher Self, journaling helps you tap into your own wisdom. Venting in your journal can be helpful as well. When I organized twenty-plus years of journals, among the jewels I wrote, I found a lot of venting that went right into the shredder. Oh yes—shredding—another stress reliever for me!

When you are overwhelmed and too busy, you may tend to either just work or just rest and leave play out of the equation. It is critical to *create play in your life!* As I write this, I remember a dream I had last night in which I arranged to no longer go into the office. I was able to set my own schedule by working from home. As soon as I realized this in the dream, I felt incredibly free and decided to walk my dog around the block and see what was around me, exploring with heightened senses. I saw myself at local coffee shops, museums, and galleries. When I awoke, I could still feel the excitement and freedom. I then realized that I have already changed my life in this way, but it subsequently just became the same daily activity of working from home. I do walk and notice what is around me and take photos, but the dream encouraged me to go to the next step, which is to drive or fly to nearby places to experience life even more ... as well as to be grateful and in the moment daily!

When you get stuck in a rut, you can focus on the same things over and over and create stress. Take some time and make plans to experience new activities that expand your senses to encompass all that you really desire.

Lastly in this list, it is important to *listen to your body and your emotions*. This is spoken about in other weeks as well. Honor yourself. One of the ways I look at how to create my life is in thinking about what age it is I will live to be. Now, you may not know, but you can make a guesstimate. I have the year in mind for myself, and I calculate how many years I have left for everything my heart desires to accomplish, experience, or travel and see. This motivates me to make plans so I don't wait too long. It is almost like a woman who has a number of remaining years in which she will be fertile and able to conceive a baby. How many years do you have left to birth your inner self?

To summarize ways in which to reduce stress, you can:

1. Compartmentalize your life—focus on one thing at a time.
2. Set realistic goals and break projects down into manageable pieces.
3. Know your limits and prioritize.
4. Eat healthy and avoid sugary snacks.
5. Decrease or alleviate caffeine altogether.
6. Move your body.
7. Get enough sleep—7 or 8 hours a night is recommended.
8. Decrease or alleviate alcohol altogether.
9. Get massage or receive healthy touch.
10. Become a non-smoker.
11. Practice relaxation.
12. Share with friends.
13. Journal.

14. Create play in your life!
15. Listen to your body and your emotions.

This is just a beginning for you to start reducing stress in your life. Often when you change your behaviors, you do not notice a difference at first. You may want to put this list on the refrigerator or a mirror and practice for six months to see how your life changes. Then assess your stress level on a scale from 1–10 again and see how much you have improved.

Tools and Exercises

I have given you some assessment tools and suggestions to help with the symptoms. Let's go a little deeper to look at possible patterns that will continue to cause stress in your life, and then we will move on to find solutions. Here are some questions for your journal:

1. Think back over the last few days. How much time was spent on high-priority activities? How much was spent on low-priority activities? What activities could have been eliminated?

2. When you needed a break, how did you handle this? Did you break and rest? Did you use food or caffeine to push through? Did you find another project that was necessary to finish? Did you find a project that was relaxing, such as cleaning out a cupboard or a drawer? Did you distract

yourself—and if so, did it have a positive or negative consequence?

3. What projects do you have that can be delegated?

4. What projects do you enjoy the most? Which are more difficult? Which do you want to avoid?

5. What time of day are you most productive? What time of day are you least productive?

6. What distracts or interrupts you the most?

I notice that when I feel stressed I have two distinct tendencies. In one, my attention on a project becomes highly focused and I micromanage the project, becoming overly focused on every detail. The other way I respond is to expand, beginning a whole new set of projects, which causes me to overwhelm myself. The overwhelming becomes a sign to refocus on completing the most important task before I begin something new.

Now, here are a few more questions for you to consider:

1. How do you behave with others when you are under stress?

2. Do you tend to say *yes* when you want to say *no*? If so, with whom do you have the most difficult time setting limits or boundaries?

3. Do you push yourself too hard? Do you have someone outside of you who pushes you to do more?

4. When you make decisions that cause others to disagree, how do you feel, and what do you do?

5. How much of your time are you spending doing what you feel you 'should' do rather than doing what you want?

6. How much of your self-esteem comes from what you produce? How comfortable are you just 'being'?

7. List the people in your life who nurture and support you. Is your primary relationship listed here?

8. How often do you set aside time to play? Who are your best play friends?

9. How much time do you spend replaying the past in your mind? Does this perhaps turn your past into your future?

10. Listen to your internal and external conversations. Do you tend to blame others, or do you take responsibility for your life?

This week brings up a lot for you to inventory and ponder. Take the time you need to do this, and be sure to return to this week as often as you need in order to move toward less stress in your life. Now, take a minute to plan a day of play in the next week!

Week Seven: Feel Your Feelings

In Week One, you evaluated your situation and looked at whether you suffer from depression or anxiety. You also read about meditation and used some tools to help you improve your situation. In Week Two, you explored how to increase passion in your life. In Week Three, you learned about food intolerance testing and how eating choices and exercise can affect your health. In Week Four, you were educated about hypnotherapy and given the opportunity to find a local hypnotherapist or practice for yourself with an online session found at my website. *(Remember to bear in mind that this is an unregulated industry. Interview the hypnotherapist for her or his level of training and experience, as well as if the two of you have a sense of rapport.)* In Week Five, you assessed your beliefs to see how they affect your feelings and health. In Week Six, you gauged your stress level and learned new solutions.

At this point, I imagine you have become aware of many thoughts and feelings. A variety of problems that underlie your pain have presented themselves, and they may be physical, emotional, mental, or even spiritual in nature. In this week, I will assist you in learning how to cope with the memories that may have surfaced, as well as the feelings and pain that accompany them.

Today, we understand that most health issues are psychologically rooted. Everything from fever blisters to cancer can be traced to emotions and beliefs. One of my favorite resources is Louise Hay, who has an incredible story about her self-healing from cancer. In her book, *Heal Your Body,* she asserts:

12 Weeks to Self-Healing

> No matter what dire their [anyone who is ill] predicament seems to be, I know that if they're willing to do the mental work of releasing and forgiving, almost anything can be healed. The word incurable, which is so frightening to so many people, really only means that the particular condition cannot be cured by "outer" methods and that we must go within to effect the healing. The condition came from nothing and will go back to nothing. [1]

Giving your attention to something you feel and believe adds energy to it. If the feelings that you experience and the thoughts you have are negative or full of anger, hate, suffering, loneliness, depression, or failure, your body will hold this information inside, and you will feel pain. If what you watch on television or read in the paper is about war and poverty, pain, anger, or riots, this becomes the metaphorical food you think about—and to which your body responds.

On the other hand, when you focus on positive thoughts and feelings such as generosity, sharing, gratitude, lovingness, and being peaceful, this also becomes metaphorical food, and your body responds to it as well. If you choose to watch television programming that is positive, read inspirational books, and search out information that is loving and from the heart, you feel better and your pain lessens. Remember, whatever you focus on increases. This dynamic is known as the Law of Attraction in metaphysical communities.

My first experience with the concept of the Law of Attraction took place when Esther and Jerry Hicks came to Spokane in the mid 1990s. If my memory serves me, they gave talks at a small church to a crowd of twenty or so and channeled a group of beings called Abraham, sharing with us through Esther Hicks. I still have the cassette tapes with all of their lessons. And then, in 2006, *The Secret* came out.[2] This movie outlines the formula for creating abundance by using the Law of Attraction.

Richard Gerber explains in his book, *Vibrational Medicine: The #1 Handbook of Subtle-Energy Therapies*, "Every atom possesses a form of consciousness," and that "when atoms of like consciousness come together and coalesce, as in the form of a crystal, there is created a body of energy which expresses a definite vibrational pattern."[3] Thus, when we create thoughts, we draw to us the same vibrational pattern created by these thoughts.

Sometimes information that is not positive is useful, especially if it motivates you to act to do something good. I watched a recorded *Oprah Winfrey* show on Earth Day. The image I saw continues to haunt me. It was a swirl of garbage sitting between the coast of California and Japan in the Pacific Ocean. The mass is ninety feet deep and the size of Texas. The garbage is killing the ocean animals and fish. This was not a positive image, but it certainly has encouraged me to recycle even more and to gently share this information with others who would be open to helping our beautiful Mother Earth heal.

Nevertheless, the feelings, thoughts, and actions that we project outward to the world are also stored in our bodies. Sometimes our bodies may be crippled from anger and fear. We may carry extra weight to protect ourselves from pain or from releasing our old pain. Maybe we have cold sores that come from stress or "burning to bitch." Once we understand how to read the body, we find ourselves to be open books. The goal is not to criticize or judge internally for having an illness, but it is to instead bring ourselves into balance. We are not just our bodies; we are physical, emotional, mental, spiritual, and social beings.

Feelings

Although much has been written about communication—between genders, parents and children, supervisors and employers, and among members of the general public—little is understood about the necessity of, and methods for, expressing feelings clearly. Most people learn to differentiate between mad, sad, glad, and scared, at best. When I hear people talk about their feelings, it is often expressed as something that happens *to* them, rather than something they notice they are experiencing from within. In this week, I focus on what appears to be the overgeneralization that fear is at the bottom of most negative feelings. Then we will explore more deeply the topic of identifying and experiencing feelings.

In metaphysical circles, the concept of feelings is often expressed as consisting of either fear or love. The goal is to move continually from fear into love as often as possible. I agree with this notion, as working on such movement is like developing a muscle that you flex. But I also think this is just another way of polarizing life by looking at situations as being either good or evil. As I noted previously, my belief is that our current experience at any given time is a process that leads us to the next process and so on, much like movie scenes lead us through the whole conceptual experience of a film.

Let's look a little closer at feelings as being similar to a muscle you flex. I see the similarity with clients often, and I remember experiencing it in my own life. It is easy to want to avoid feeling, because you may spontaneously feel overwhelmed with emotion, and then sadness or depression comes over you, which might take days or more to subside. Yet what you will learn through practice is to feel the feeling, and let it go quickly. A sad feeling can last a few minutes, and then you return to joy once you learn to feel the pure feeling and let it go. Much as you would flex a muscle and then let it go, you will learn to feel the feeling and let it go.

I know this may sound difficult, but I have experienced this dynamic often, even after having spent my twenties and thirties crying in bed for days. What I like to say to clients is, "Feel your feelings, and they will go away." Today, most often when I am sad or cry, it comes over me like a wave, and I have no idea what has brought it on. I have already cleared the stories attached to the feeling, so when a feeling arises now, it is usually triggered by a movie or someone else's story. It comes over me, I cry deeply for a moment, and it is gone. I don't try to figure out what it was about or why I felt the feelings—none of that. I just thank God (you can thank whatever Higher Power to which you connect, including God, Goddess, Universe, etc.) for that healing, and I go on. Note here that I see the feeling as a healing, because that is truly what it is. Again, while this might seem difficult now, trust in the process.

I spoke about William Glasser and cognitive therapy in Week One. The way he describes feelings is that we experience a pure feeling, which lasts for three to ten seconds, and then it is gone. However, what we often do is attach a story to the feeling, and then the feeling can last for years.

To demonstrate this, you can imagine watching a young child fall. For example, I watch my 22-month-old granddaughter. She hits the ground and immediately takes stock of what's happened. If I run to her in reaction, she will cry. But I find if I am neutral and just watch her, she assesses the situation and goes on. This happened last week when we were walking a trail by the Spokane River. She was walking fast, grasping to get her stride down a slope of the trail that is full of small rocks. I attempted to hold her hand, but she told me not to do so. Next, she tumbled and was on her knees and little hands. She looked shocked at first but then carefully lifted one of her hands and looked at it. "Dirty!" she exclaimed as she saw the dirt stuck to her palms. I walked over to her and told her to wipe the dirt on Grandma's pants, and she was as happy as could be. Off she went to find the big rock pile. I am sure you have noticed this with your own loved ones.

Earlier I used the words *feelings* and *emotions* interchangeably, but let's look at those words. In her 2000 book, *Feelings Buried Alive Never Die*, Karol K. Truman differentiates between the two. She writes:

> If you became very angry at someone but held the anger inside—this is a FEELING. However, if you became angry and let yourself explode, either verbally or physically, the feeling of anger would then be manifesting itself as an EMOTION. In other words, the emotion is the outward expression or reaction of the FEELING. Or ... the EMOTION is the result of a thought and an intense feeling coming together.[4]

The way I understand this is that if you don't experience your feelings—if you don't feel them and let them go away—you can go from having an angry feeling to being an angry person.

Thanks to Einstein, other scientists, and those who study quantum physics, we know that everything is made of energy. We know that all life forms are energy, and we know that even rocks, plants, and the bed on which you sleep are energy. We also know that energy cannot be destroyed, but it can be transformed. All of your body is energy, from the follicles in your hair to the nails on your toes. It is all energy in motion.

It is also true that your feelings and your thoughts are energy. Truman writes that thoughts and feelings are energy.[5] They are atoms composed of tiny amounts of pure energy, better described as waves of energy solidified or frozen into the non-movement recognized as matter. Matter is a form of energy that is in very slow or stopped motion (or frequency). Since matter cannot be destroyed, but can be altered, you can change your feeling or thought that is negative matter (energy) into positive matter (energy). Truman espouses the idea that a feeling or thought becomes a negative energy when it obscures the truth of our Being. We are all a reflection of the Universe and of universal love. This is what you want to remember and hold as your focus.

When I was studying religion as an undergraduate student, what I determined for myself was that sin was whatever took us away from our true connection with Spirit, God, or in this case, with our own perfect Being. Truman continued to explore the notion of thoughts and feelings as energy.

Energy travels at the rate of 186,000 miles per second. This means thought can travel 186,000 miles per second also ... or faster. Energy moves in pulses—like waves. The crest is the pulse of energy and the thought is the pause. How close together the waves are is called frequencies—how frequently the waves occur. This range of frequencies is called the electro-magnetic spectrum. What we see, feel and experience materially is but a tiny part of the entire electro-magnetic spectrum. ... All elements of the earth have different energies. ... The closer together the vibrational frequencies, the higher the vibration and the closer that matter is to its energy Source. ... Likewise, the more broad the frequencies of any given matter, the further that energy is from its Source.[6]

Bruce Lipton, in *The Biology of Belief*, argued that our feelings and beliefs are hard-wired in our DNA. He asserted that:

The fundamental behaviors, beliefs and attitudes we observe in our parents become "hard-wired" as synaptic pathways in our subconscious minds. Once programmed into the subconscious mind, they control our biology for the rest of our lives ... unless we can figure out a way to reprogram them.[7]

Lipton further suggested that electroencephalograms (EEGs) show variations in frequency in the brain, from low frequency delta waves to high frequency beta waves.[8] Research has shown that these frequencies change with developmental ages. Lipton cites Dr. Rima Laibow, in *Quantitative EEG and Neurofeedback*, as explaining that between birth and age two, the predominant frequency is 0.5 to 4 cycles per second (Hz).[9] This is the delta wave. Although babies have spurts of higher frequency, they do not move to the higher theta level of 4–8 Hz until two to six years of age. The lower frequencies of these two brain states allow for a more suggestible and programmable condition. This is the reason children learn so much so quickly, as well as the reason that hypnotherapists use these states to help reprogram clients into achieving goals.

With age, the frequency increases to alpha waves, 8–12 Hz, which is a calm state of consciousness.[10] In this state, one becomes more aware of self and is not as programmable by the outside environment. Around age twelve, the frequency increases to 12–35 Hz, and the consciousness is more focused and active, such as that employed when reading a book.[11] A higher state of EEG frequency is the gamma wave state, which is > 35 Hz. This frequency is connected to peak performance, such as the level of consciousness needed to land a plane or play professional tennis.[12]

Lipton talks about the two minds we have: the conscious mind and the subconscious mind. The programming learned as a young person, the feelings that are "hard-wired," come from the subconscious mind.[13] Therefore, although people have free will, in order to change the programming, an individual would need to become fully conscious about the programming to do so.

It is fascinating that the conscious mind can think forward and backward in time, but the subconscious mind is always in present time. Though you may have great plans for something (conscious mind), you may find yourself doing different behaviors or having different feelings than expected (programmed subconscious mind). This dynamic can show up in the learned behaviors and beliefs that were acquired from others but no longer support the conscious beliefs you have today.

Lipton describes the subconscious as "an emotionless database of stored programs, whose function is strictly concerned with reading environmental signals and engaging in hard-wired behavioral programs."[14] The problem here is that these "programmed reflexes" have you reacting to a situation the way you did when you first learned this behavior; thus you find yourself "getting your buttons pushed." In her book, *Anatomy of the Spirit*, Caroline Myss talks about this programmed information, calling it tribal information that is located in the first chakra.[15] This concept will be explored in Week Seven when I outline and discuss the chakras in greater detail.

I just completed a session in Kyoto with a beautiful young woman whose father owns a hospital. She has been working for her family and wants to do something else, but in Japan, they are most often true to the group and not as individual as we are in the West. She began to cry as she explained that when her mother was pregnant with her, her father was having an affair. Although my agent was translating, it was not hard to see the pain in the young woman's heart, and I felt the affinity of all women as she shared. The story that her mother told was that she was sad, and the client declared that she remembered this feeling in the womb and that it had resulted in her being born with the following belief: "I should not exist."

Her remembrance is not an isolated case. I find similar memories in myself and most of my clients. Although we may not have rational thoughts at that point in our existence, we do have feelings, and I believe we also have subconscious *knowingness*. When we are in our mother's womb and during the birthing process, we have an experience that sets the stage for our beliefs. Our beliefs then become a filter for our view of the world, and if there is information in the world that does not fit in our belief system, we choose not to allow this information in. Our Ego continues to support our belief system, and therefore whatever we believe is what appears to us to be true. We then go on to defend this belief in our need to be right— even if the belief, as in the example above, is painful and self-effacing.

I have been trained in eye movement desensitization and reprocessing (EMDR), so I used this process and was able to help the young woman clear her erroneous and damaging belief and replace it with the following: "I appreciate being born, and I love life."[16] I was so happy to see the expression on her face change from one of despair to one of hope as she left the session.

I have been assisting clients in clearing negative energy, as well as identifying and replacing beliefs, for many years. My first experience with clearing energy began with Mary Ellen Flora's work and the Church of Divine Man. Flora demonstrates using the Creating and Destroying Roses Technique in her 2002 book, *Healing: Key to Spiritual Balance.*[17] In May of 2000, I took a class on DNA reprocessing and repatterning.[18] In this class, we learned to identify the matrix of beliefs that we hold and to clear the negative beliefs from the DNA, replacing them with positive beliefs. This teaching was on the cutting edge of healing in working with virtual strands of DNA.

During the class, I remember working my own health issue; I had held pain in my lower back for several months and was experiencing it at the workshop. The underlying belief I had derived was that "being in a body sucks." As you can imagine, the major feeling I had was anger. My workshop partner and I went through the process in the book and replaced this belief with the following: "I am happy, healthy, and love my body." My pain was released immediately, and I didn't experience this pain again on a regular basis. This was an incredible, prayerful process that I have continued to use in my private practice. Some other examples are to clear fear of being controlled and replace it with being in balanced control of self, to clear fear of living/dying and replace it with love of life, and to clear fear of being too fat or too thin and replace it with perfect metabolism.

More recently, I completed Part I and Part II in the eye movement desensitization and reprocessing (EMDR) class. This class is offered only to master's level and higher practitioners and is accepted by the American Psychological Association (APA). This process is similar to the one I speak of in the preceding paragraph, in that both identify the underlying beliefs of illness, clear the beliefs, and install a new, healthy belief. EMDR is defined on the EMDR website, **http://www.emdr.com**, as an information processing therapy. There is a protocol in which the client identifies the trauma, addresses the underlying belief, and creates a new belief that is installed by the use of the eye movement or pulsers. The client is also able to clear the emotional charge and where that charge is stored in the body. This process is highly successful in treating trauma.

On my way to Missoula, Montana for the EMDR training workshop from Spokane, I drove over the Fourth of July Pass (in Idaho). I don't like driving near semis, so I sped up my little car and whipped around in order to not be near them. I soon learned that this was not the smartest plan. Although these large trucks were slow and dragging on the uphill, on the downslope I had five semis right behind me, coming down fast. I panicked and could barely stay on the road because I was so scared. When I got to the workshop, I used this as my first issue to clear. As was described earlier, I was in a car accident when I was fourteen years old and ended up thrown from the vehicle. In the course of the EMDR processing, I realized the semis triggered this old fear response. We cleared this, and on the trip back home I was fine!

Beliefs are created by your experiences in life, your culture, as well as what you have heard, read, and seen. Beliefs are not facts, but they may feel like facts. Because of the many years of practice and different methods used in clearing outdated beliefs or ones that didn't serve me, in my intuitive coaching practice, I now see how empowered clients are when they identify the belief systems that have kept them stuck or unable to create the life of their dreams.

The sources cited throughout this week may prove helpful if you would like to explore more about how to change beliefs. To assist you in clearing beliefs, I have developed my own system, which is a combination of tools I have used for years and find particularly effective. I invite you to participate in the following exercise:

Write out a specific situation that is painful for you. Allow yourself to be detailed and use the writing process as a therapeutic tool. This gets the "charge" up on the situation. Then pick out the **main issue** you have with the situation and list it.

1. Write out the belief related to this situation. The way to determine this is to ask yourself, "What decision did I make about myself regarding this situation?" It usually starts with "I am" and is the **core belief** you will be replacing.

2. Decide upon the **new belief** you want to create and use as a replacement. Write this new belief down.

3. Now, focus in your heart. Bring your consciousness up into the heavens. Ask to connect with your Source or to whomever you pray. Ask Source to clear the core belief at the core past/present/future. Image this belief dissolving.

Image golden white light swirling and clearing the core belief. Take a deep breath from your belly and let it out. Focus in your heart. Now, take the new belief you want to create. Bring your consciousness up into the heavens and see yourself living, experiencing, and feeling this new belief. Use all of your senses. Feel yourself swirling in golden-white light, and bring this belief down through the top of your head, filling your whole body with this belief. Ground your energy. Focus in your heart and thank your Source for this healing. It is done, it is done, it is done.

Prior to clearing and replacing beliefs, you may want to use the Comparative Pain Scale from the first week to assess your pain level prior to and after the clearing. Keep notes in your journal so that you can check back in a month or so in order to see whether these issues have cleared or whether other issues relevant to the first one have surfaced.

I was traveling in London last year, schlepping my luggage up and down the stairs of the Tube and my hotel in Notting Hill. In this process, I pulled or tore something in my right shoulder or arm. Over the last year, the pain moved a lot, so I was unsure about where the original damage had been. I didn't do much about it and thought it would just go away if I didn't move it a great deal. But being the grandmother of a growing toddler, I kept reinjuring myself in picking her up or throwing her a ball. I decided to get massage for it on a regular basis. The massage therapist told me if I didn't start moving the shoulder, it would become frozen, and she gave me some exercises to do.

Then I decided to go to Dr. Patrick Dougherty, a chiropractor I know who uses kinesiology and works on a spiritual level as well. He worked on my body in the first session, and I felt much better. In the second session, he began working on my belief system. He used a process of muscle testing, which is also kinesiology, and identified a belief of mine.

At the time I could only move my arm up from my side at about twenty-five percent of my normal range of motion. After having me look through a set of different colored glasses (literally), with kinesiology, he chose the glasses that corresponded with the heart chakra. This identified the chakra where the belief was stored that affected my arm movement. He then identified the pertinent belief from a list he had outlined in a notebook and asked me to repeat, "I am not affected by the lack of compassion in the world." When he used kinesiology, I tested weak, meaning the statement was not true; I *was* affected by the lack of compassion. He then cleared this belief by tapping on my spine a couple of times. After he had done so, I could move my arm at fifty percent of my normal range of motion. It was clear that it was important for me to acknowledge how the lack of compassion in the world bothers me. I was amazed! Even though clearing beliefs and working with healing through belief systems is the same work I have been doing for fifteen years, it was still incredible to be the recipient of this healing.

When working with clients using DNA reprocessing and repatterning, I ask them to tell me what was happening at the time they were born. I inquire about what the relationship was like between their parents, whether or not there were siblings, what their parents were doing for work, where they were living, and if their parents were happy at the time. I ask for any stories they've heard about their parents' lives during that time. I also ask what the birth was like for the mother. Often in this process, I hear very significant information that affected the client's life for years.

I actually remember doing this process myself when I first learned it. When I took myself back to the womb, I remember thinking about my parents' situation prior to my actual birth. The thought I had was, "This is a mess, but I can fix it." That became my main belief in life, and yes, my life became about fixing my family. I continued to act according to this belief as a chemical dependency counselor, and then a mental health counselor, and then a healer, a teacher of spiritual healing, and then a writer. The difference is that through healing, my position changed from one of fixing to one of empowering.

The purpose of this section is to help you understand how closely aligned your feelings are with your beliefs, and how beliefs happen at a very early age and carry on through your life. When I took the class on DNA reprocessing and repatterning, the way this was explained is that you have a matrix of lines around you, each representing a belief. Your beliefs can be about religion, food, gender, politics, values—all of the beliefs you may have. You are generally not conscious of these beliefs, and yet they govern your life. Remember the conscious and subconscious mind discussed previously. The goal is to identify and replace the beliefs that no longer serve you. So, as you move into the actual feelings themselves, please be aware of the beliefs you have beneath the feelings.

Some of the beliefs and replacement beliefs I have worked with are listed here:

"I am unworthy,"	replaced with:	"I am worthy."
"I am undeserving,"	replaced with:	"I deserve love."
"I am helpless,"	replaced with:	"I forgive myself and will not put other's interests before my own."
"No one takes me seriously,"	replaced with:	"What I say is important."
"I am not supported,"	replaced with:	"I am strong and I accept support."
"I don't trust my judgment,"	replaced with:	"I trust myself."
"I am unlovable,"	replaced with:	"I am lovable."

These are beliefs underlying the situations in which clients find themselves, and they are similar to those we all experience with family, work, or in social situations. In addition to identifying the beliefs with my clients, we also identify the feelings. That being said, many people cannot identify what they are feeling. Let's continue this week by exploring some common feelings. Later in this week we will look at communication and identify the difference between thoughts and feelings.

Now that you have this information about beliefs and feelings being hard-wired, how can you better identify and replace the beliefs? What happens when you are overwhelmed with feelings? Let's start with fear.

Fear

Fear is a feeling that can be motivating—and paralyzing. If you feel fearful when passing a car on the freeway near a bend in the road, the feeling may help you stay safe. If you are fearful for no particular reason about leaving your home, the fear is irrational and most likely will have underlying beliefs attached. Some of the symptoms of fear are tightness in the throat and chest, lack of energy, trouble breathing, dry mouth, weakness in the muscles, a hollow feeling in your gut, and oversensitivity to movement and noise.

Behaviors that are related to fear are as follows:

1. Being unable to sleep, oversleeping, or sleeping restlessly.
2. Overeating or lack of appetite.
3. Withdrawing socially, not engaging in activities or isolating.
4. Crying.
5. Being absentminded.
6. Being restless or engaging in overactivity.
7. Clinging to memories or treasured items.

Overcoming fear tends to be difficult for many people. It often gets buried underneath anger or another emotion. To overcome the fear, try the following options:

1. Begin a meditation practice as described in Week Eight. Meditation is an excellent deterrent to feeling fear.

2. Use self-hypnosis. When you take yourself into a trance with the intention of feeling confident and secure, your subconscious will naturally work with you to overcome the fear. The more often you practice this, the better.

3. Challenge your thoughts. This is another helpful way to overcome the fear. Use the technique outlined for this in the Tools and Exercises section at the end of this week.

4. Look at the belief underneath this fear and clear the belief, as I described just a bit ago.

5. Remember, what you focus on increases. Distract yourself, focus on something else, and continue to do what evokes the fear. An example of this for me is the way I handle my needle phobia. When I have to get a shot or a test, I close my eyes, create an image of my granddaughter, and focus on her. Before I know it, I am ready to leave.

Anger

It is natural to feel angry at times. It is important to recognize when you feel angry and be able to resolve the feelings. In this section, we will look at positive ways to express your feelings of anger. It is helpful to know that anger is a secondary emotion. Underneath anger is pain and fear.

There are three basic ways of expressing anger that are generally not effective. Some people feel the anger and are explosive. Others are passive-aggressive and avoid direct contact, instead seeking revenge or punishing others by behaving like martyrs. They may also express the anger with verbal abuse. The third type of expression is stuffing the anger. In this case, people punish themselves and turn anger inward rather than outward. This expression of anger can take place through self-destructive measures and self-sabotage.

Information about communication and learning to identify feelings clearly will be addressed later in the book, but in this section I will help you to identify the anger symptoms and learn some tools to help you release the anger.

It is helpful to be able to identify the way you respond to anger in your mind and your body. Some of these responses are as follows:

1. Your mind races and you have negative, angry, or abusive thoughts.

2. Your muscles tense, especially in your neck and face.

3. You feel hot or cold.

4. Your breathing increases.

5. Your temperature rises.

6. You feel like yelling or screaming.

7. You grit your teeth.

8. Your hands become fists.

9. Your stomach hurts or churns.

10. You want to move, walk, stomp, or kick something.

11. Adrenaline increases in your body and you feel a sense of power.

When you feel angry, you may exhibit the following behaviors:

1. You explode at the person with whom you are angry.

2. You become angry and verbal with those who are not directly related to the situation. This may be the person on the other end of the phone when you are attempting to straighten out an error on a phone bill, or it could be the person in the car who just pulled out in front of you.

3. You make rude comments to or about others under your breath.

4. You find yourself complaining about others behind their back or in your mind.

5. You choose to withdraw from others.

6. You don't complete assignments, or you do them poorly.

7. You start rebelling about rules and challenge them for no apparent reason.

Think for a moment about how you deal with your anger. You may have developed some positive ways to handle it. In my private practice, I have seen over the years that when clients were angry, they often reverted to the methods they learned when they were children. Here are some constructive ways to channel your anger. Remember that when you feel your feelings, they go away.

1. It would first be good for you to journal and see if you can find out what is underneath the anger. You may write about what scares you. Next, write out what is painful or who may have hurt your feelings.

2. If you are in a situation in which you or the other person may get out of control, walk away. Angry outbursts are not rational, and you are likely to regret it if you stay and allow the irrational feelings to become irrational behavior.

3. Your mind will probably be racing, so if you can, start to move your body. Go for a brisk walk, get on your bike, or shoot some hoops.

4. Pick up your journal and write an angry letter. This venting can really help.

5. Vent to a friend. Be careful to talk with a friend who can remain neutral and not take sides in the interest of not damaging any of your relationships in the future.

6. Dialogue with yourself. Why did this person or situation trigger you? Underneath anger is most

likely pain or fear. How did this situation hurt you? What are you afraid of?

7. Breathe! Take a few deep breaths. Breathe in to the count of seven and breathe out to the count of eleven. Do this until your body is calm.

8. Change the image in your mind. Focus on something that gives you joy. Think of your child, grandchild, spouse, a trip coming up, or your pet.

You can go back later and analyze what belief was triggered. Once you identify it, use the information and process I've provided above regarding changing your beliefs. Remember, your feelings come from what you are thinking. You are in control!

Throughout this book, I refer to managing your pain. Walking down the street in Kyoto one morning, looking for Keihan Fushimi Inari station, I became aware of how we make choices, and how these choices come from beliefs that affect feelings and the physical body. After seeing clients one day and facilitating a two-day meditation workshop at the Fushini Inari Shrine, I found myself carrying a heavy physical load. My neck began to ache, and my back joined in as I carried a purse full of necessities and a backpack with my computer and books.

In going to Japan, I had made the choice to honor a previously planned business trip at the same time I was headed for an important writing deadline. Of course, the increased pressure added to my stress. This schedule was my choice, and I had to take responsibility for how it would affect my body. You may be able to relate to this. When you are honest with yourself, you can process your thoughts and feelings and not store the pain deep in your body; instead, you deal with it in present time. With practice, it becomes easier to own a choice involving behavior. While it is not as easy to see, you also choose your feelings.

Grief

As I said before, when we feel our feelings, they go away. This statement refers to experiencing pure feeling, not replaying all the stories we attach to the feelings. Grief comes in waves. Often, what you have not healed completely will attach to a recent grief. For example, say a dear friend passes on. You may feel the loss of this friend while also experiencing grief over another loved one whom you lost many years before. What I often find when counseling clients is that loss is frequently not only about losing people but also about choices or opportunities not taken. Sometimes you may have forgotten that you once had a plan for your life that you didn't manifest, and this loss has gone underground and caused a low-grade depression.

Several years ago, I was counseling a man who shared that he and his wife had saved money for years so they could travel after retirement. They had planned to go to Switzerland, which was the home of his ancestors. The couple had watched videos, read books, and visualized themselves there often. Then the wife came down with cancer and was not able to travel. While she could not be that far from home, the couple had adult children who could care for her. My client was disappointed and sad. In our counseling sessions, it became clear that he really wanted and needed to allow himself to go to Switzerland. He said his wife agreed with this, but he felt sad that she couldn't go, adding that he would feel guilty if he went. This was a dilemma for him. If he didn't go, he would regret it and grieve for a potentially long time. If he did go, he would need to give himself full permission to do so, or else he would "guilt himself" for years. I never did find out what decision he made, but I hope it was the one that gave him joy.

Guilt

Guilt is an interesting feeling. The value of guilt is that you can use it to stop yourself from doing behaviors that are hurtful to yourself or others. My experience is that guilt also becomes a tool of control. Too many times it is used to manipulate others in an attempt to control them. You may make others feel bad about what they do, or you may self-punish with guilt. Even if you are not actually hurting yourself or others, this emotion still tends to be overused and unhelpful. In my private practice, I often help clients drop guilt in order give themselves permission for any number of things.

Parents often say no to protect a child, but I find in the American culture that often parents say no because they are tired or overworked, and it is easier to say no than to take the time to listen to a child or plan an activity. If you heard "no" often as a child, there is an interject, which means your parents' voices live on in your head. What I usually say is, "You swallowed your parent, and the voice continues." When these children become adults, often they do not allow themselves simple pleasures, because their heads are full of "no." They feel guilty when they are generous with themselves, or they just feel guilty for no known reason.

Of course, balance is important. If you tend to deny yourself, it is helpful to give yourself permission more often. If you don't set boundaries with yourself, then of course staying on track and setting boundaries will be helpful. Whether you struggle with rigidity toward yourself or a lack of boundaries, the situation can create problems with your thinking, beliefs, and health.

Boundaries

Whether you are male or female, young or old, it is often difficult to set appropriate boundaries. There are the boundaries you set within yourself and the ones you set outside yourself. Setting a boundary within may be setting a boundary of discipline. For instance, let's say you are studying for an exam, and your friend calls to say she has two tickets to a music concert. You really want to go, but you know that you will not be able to study for the exam if you see the concert. The internal boundary would be to say no.

I will offer you another example of an internal boundary. You have a friend who is pregnant. You had a difficult experience giving birth. You know that it will be helpful for you to talk about it, but you also know it would not be kind to share this information with your friend. You set the internal boundary to keep this information to yourself and listen to your friend's experience while later journaling about your experience or talking with another friend.

An example of setting a boundary outside yourself might be the experience of a friend coming to visit when you have several projects to complete before you can give your friend your full attention. Then your daughter calls and asks if you will babysit for a few hours. She tells you she has an opportunity to go to a special event, and there is no one else available. Although you love your beautiful grandchild, you know that you will not be able to get your projects done with a toddler near. Nevertheless, you say *yes*, giving up your own needs. Later you find yourself exhausted and in pain from pushing so hard to complete your projects, as well as really angry with yourself. One option may be to blame your daughter, but the reality is that we make choices and then experience the consequences. Blaming anger on others and continuing this resentment can easily turn into physical pain

Anger is such a good teacher, and it helps us learn to set a boundary. Imagine the above scenario. Imagine that, instead of saying yes to your daughter, you set a boundary around your time and needs. This decision results in maintaining your energy and your health, and you feel empowered. When you are first learning to set internal boundaries, it is likely to take some practice. Similarly, setting external boundaries may feel unfamiliar, and you may fear that those with whom you set boundaries will reject you, or you may feel guilty. With practice, you will feel empowered and may realize how easy it is for others to adjust to your limits and requests for your own space and time.

It is important to listen to your own needs, especially when suffering from pain. You're giving away your precious energy when you don't set boundaries. If you say *yes* when really thinking *no*, it affects your health. (This is generally a third chakra issue. We'll explore this more fully in an upcoming week.) Your self-esteem is affected by the choices you make. Below, boundaries are discussed in terms of being collapsed, rigid, or healthy.

Collapsed Boundaries

When boundaries are collapsed, the tendency is to say *yes* when you want to say *no*, as we just discussed. In this case, you often do not even know that you don't want to agree to whatever is on the other end, because the habit of accommodating others has become so engrained. Examples of this would be parents who give in to their children when asked for money, a cell phone—or even to babysit later on in life—when they would prefer to say *no*. They may fear their children will be angry with them or abandon and reject them, so they continue to give in.

If you have people in your life who really do reject or abandon you when you set limits, this is known as being "taken hostage." They control you through giving or taking away love. While we've already learned that you cannot be controlled and that you are in control of what you feel, it is not always easy to live in a way that reflects this knowledge. This book offers you some tools for learning to separate yourself enough to feel empowered by your own thoughts and decisions, rather than by those of others.

We all know the person who always agrees to help when it comes to volunteering. You may be this person. There is a need at the school or neighborhood committee meeting, and the same person is always doing more than his or her fair share. This may be a collapsed boundary. When you begin to say *no* after having said *yes* for years, you often feel guilty or fearful, but this continued giving when it is not right for your own needs or inner self is depleting. It takes a toll on your health.

Another example of a collapsed boundary is sharing too much information too soon. You may meet someone for the first time and hear that person's life history or simply more than you care to know. You may feel uncomfortable with all of the personal information and not know how to respond. If your own boundaries are collapsed, you may take on the person's feelings as your own. You may even respond by fixing, rescuing, or problem solving for that person.

Taking on other people's feelings happens often in families. A wife may not know what she feels apart from her husband or her children. A coworker may take on the stress of his boss or partner and cease being able to discern his own feelings. By now you have hopefully started using the journal process. It is helpful to journal in order to get clear on your responsibility, what you feel, and what belongs to the other person with respect to stress, feelings, and responsibilities.

Another sample of collapsed boundaries is avoiding conflict. It is often difficult to share what you are feeling with someone whose reaction in the past has been anger. It sometimes seems easier to just not say anything—and the reality is, at times this is true. The important thing to discern here is the difference between what needs to be discussed and what you can let go. There are times when what you have to say is really important, and being honest is a matter of integrity. At these times, avoiding conflict is not the answer. Conflict can result in bringing up issues that need to be addressed, and when you avoid the issue, the feelings you have attached to the issue become buried. The problem is that they are buried alive, and they will surface again when you least expect them, sometimes creating embarrassing situations. They may also go dormant and begin to affect your health. The energy gets stuck in your auric field or your biofield (a low-level electromagnetic field produced by the human body) and shuts down your body's ability to clear itself and self-heal.

People with collapsed boundaries often lack a sense of self. Their ideas and opinions are not their own, but they take on the ideas and opinions of others. I have seen this often in young women who have aligned themselves with something that is more powerful than they are, such as a boyfriend or the beliefs of a church or political group. Temporarily this can be helpful, but at some point they need to emancipate and learn to know themselves. I have seen many people who've felt lost or weak align with a fundamentalist church of some type, gang, or other group that views life in black-and-white terms. This gives the person who feels lost or weak a set of absolute rules for living. When I refer to a black-and-white thinking group, I am referring to people who see the world in terms of extremes. There is little gray area or room for individual perception. Some political and religious groups have had devastating effects on those who've followed them blindly.

Similarly, there are people who are not able to figure out who they are because they have learned to behave the way others want them to behave. They become predictable, and often the people they are attempting to please get bored with or weary of them. This sends them into crisis, which is often of a medical or emotional nature. Although taking time to find out who you are and what you believe may seem like a luxury to some of us, to these people it is terrifying.

Those who have collapsed boundaries frequently have a high tolerance for abuse and are able to live with disrespect for long periods. I had a male client, Sean, who came to see me because his wife, Shauna, told him he was "controlling." She became depressed and felt suicidal, and he was devastated and wanted to find out how to help her. I immediately noticed a sign of collapsed boundaries as Sean sat forward in his seat, decreasing the distance between us by over a foot. This is a red flag to counselors suggesting that boundary issues will need to be addressed.

Sean and I met for a couple of sessions before I gave him Melody Beattie's book, *Codependent No More*.[19] Sean said he really enjoyed the book; it had helped a lot, and he had even purchased it for some friends. We worked with this view of his being codependent for a few sessions, until he disclosed the rest of the story. He and his wife Shauna were friends with another couple. Nathan, the husband of the other couple, was spending a lot of time with Shauna while Sean was at work. In fact, Nathan set Shauna up in a business in which they worked together for hours during the daytime when Sean was at work, and even at night when Sean came home. Sean told Nathan and Shauna straightforwardly that he was concerned about their relationship. Nathan assured Sean that, even though he loved her, they were not "doing anything" and that his time spent with Shauna was necessary in order for her to get well. As the story went on, it became clear that Nathan and Shauna were having some kind of intimate relationship that was destructive to Sean and Shauna's marriage and to their physical health as well.

As we explored the situation more, it became clear to Sean that he needed to confront his wife and set a boundary around her relationship with Nathan. Sean had lived with this situation for years and definitely had a high tolerance for disrespect and subtle abuse. He finally did confront his wife, and she agreed that she would not see Nathan. The friendship ended, and Shauna started going to counseling to work through the affair she had been having. Sean was empowered by confronting the situation and came through it feeling good about standing up for himself and saving his marriage.

Sometimes when you are abused or neglected in a relationship, you feel as if you deserve the treatment you have received. You take responsibility for what happened. I believe part of this is due to an attempt at having some control. If you take responsibility and consider it to be your fault, then you feel in control. If it is the other person's fault, you feel powerless. This reasoning comes from low self-esteem and often a history of neglect or abuse in the past, or from witnessing this pattern as a child.

Rigid Boundaries

Rather than having boundaries that are too weak, some people have rigid boundaries that keep everyone at a distance. When you have rigid boundaries, you may keep to yourself and not connect well with others. You may automatically say no to a request if this request would involve close interaction. This of course is a simple understanding of boundaries and does not take into account social anxiety and phobias.

Another way you might exhibit rigid boundaries is by having strong defenses to protect yourself from being close to others. This could show up as you being defensive and prickly or not easy to be around. It could also show up as being argumentative, which keeps others away. Staying busy and not having time for friends or loved ones is another example of behavior that accompanies rigid boundaries.

I have seen this often with clients who are going through divorce. Initially the distance between the two individuals is okay because they both have their own full lives. As the marriage develops, many of the activities and friends become commingled. Then, if one partner has rigid boundaries, that person stops attending the parties or activities or stays late at work, and he or she drops out of the communal marriage. Eventually the two people grow apart as the one partner longs for closeness, and the other is comfortable being isolated.

Fear can contribute to rigid boundaries if you are afraid of abandonment or engulfment. You may want to connect deeply, but if you have had experiences of being left behind as a child or in previous relationships, you may not dare to let anyone get close. On the flip side, rigid boundaries can be established due to fear of being taken over by (or losing yourself in) another person. If a parent or other relative was smothering during your childhood, and if they lived their life through you or were very controlling, you may create distance in order to avoid emotional hurt, or in order to maintain a sense of self. This can also be the case if you experienced a lack of boundaries or collapsed boundaries in an early love relationship. Creating distance can provide a sense of safety.

You will notice that some people disclose a lot about themselves, while others make little or no self-disclosure. People who have rigid boundaries may talk easily and draw the other person out, but not share about themselves. This often leaves the person who has shared freely feeling as if she or he has over-disclosed at the end of the conversation. This lack of self-disclosure can lead a person to have an inability to identify her or his own wants, needs, and feelings, which can create problems in a relationship, especially if one partner has collapsed boundaries and the other has rigid boundaries. You will notice that someone who has rigid boundaries will have several acquaintances, but few close friends. I see this often in my private practice, especially among women. They are beautiful, accomplished women who do well professionally, but have few to no friends.

Healthy Boundaries

Now that we have identified the characteristics of collapsed and rigid boundaries, let's explore what it looks like to have healthy boundaries. When you have healthy boundaries, you are able to say *no* to a request, and to say *yes* as well. You are able to communicate clearly when you feel that someone is pressuring you or encroaching on your territory. You are also able to hear *no* from others and seek other resources to get your needs met. It is not clear whether strong boundaries or healthy self-esteem comes first, but when you have healthy boundaries, you have a strong sense of identity and self-respect. Likewise, when you have a strong sense of identity and a healthy self-respect, you set appropriate boundaries.

When you have healthy boundaries, you reveal information about yourself gradually and self-disclose in an appropriate manner. Relationships feel more balanced, and there is an expectation of sharing responsibility for the relationship. When appropriate boundaries have been set, it is easier to discern whether a problem is yours, whether it belongs to the other person, or whether it is a mutual issue. There is little blaming when you take responsibility for yourself in a relationship. You also honor the other person's ability to conduct proper self-care and do not tend to jump in to rescue the individual. You may lend a helping hand if it is appropriate to do so, but for the most part, you recognize that the person is the best candidate to solve his or her own problems. When you have a healthy boundary, you do not tolerate disrespect or abuse and can communicate directly and clearly—and leave if necessary.

Communication

Now that we have identified the differences between collapsed, rigid, and healthy boundaries, let's look at communication. If you have not identified your particular patterns around boundaries, it may be helpful to do so before moving on to communication. This is a general overview to give you some tools to increase your success at communicating and being heard or understood.

It is difficult to address communication with others without talking about communication with yourself. The first step in communication is being clear with yourself about what it is you want to convey to the other person. It is also important to be aware of how well you listen to others. It may be helpful for you to make notes in your journal as you remember times when communication has been difficult in the past, so that you can assess what happened and move to resolve the pattern in order to ensure it will not be repeated. Since this book is about self-healing and emotional and physical pain, we will focus primarily on communication with those who are most involved in your life. They may include your parents, children, friends, caregivers, and professionals who are involved in your care, such as your doctor, acupuncturist, or therapist.

We have already addressed beliefs and self-talk. Assuming you've identified some of these patterns, let's look next at how you communicate with others. Some people generally use direct communication, while others use indirect communication. *Direct communication* is authoritative; you usually know what the person wants, and little discussion is required. It also usually directs action. If she is using an authoritative style, your daughter may say to you, "Mom, I'll pick you up at three o'clock to take you to the market." *Indirect communication* usually elicits input or a response from someone else. Instead of being authoritative, it is more passive. If she is speaking indirectly, your daughter may say, "Mom, I am available if you need a ride to the market."

In some cases, indirect communication can also be confusing. For example, you may wish your daughter would take you to the market because you are running out of groceries. However, you know that she is busy and in a hurry, so when she asks if you need to go to the market, you reply, "Oh, I'm fine. I have enough groceries." She will not know what you really need. If it turns out that you went without important things, you may feel resentful, and if your daughter finds out, she may feel guilty. This is why it is important for you to know what you really want and be able to ask for it. If you were to say, "Are you going to the store soon?" you would still be using indirect communication, but at least it would imply a need on your part. The result might very well be that your daughter would arrange to get you to the market or pick up groceries for you as the result of a communicative process.

When communicating, it is important to have a win-win intention. In this mode, you are able to express what you need, and the other person is able to hear what you are communicating. We discussed some of this in the section on feelings. When you don't communicate clearly, or when you don't get your needs met, resentment tends to grow, and this can settle in your body as pain or illness.

I particularly like the way communication is described in the Essential Peacemaking: Women and Men program I facilitated in the nineties.[20] In this program, communication was described as either collaborative communication or defensive communication. *Collaborative communication* happens when you are interested in your own truth and the truth of the other person. In this style of communication, you are just as interested in the other person's needs as you are in your own. You listen to know the person better and to understand that you are hearing him or her correctly. This is listening with your heart. At times, you may lovingly interrupt to make sure you are able to understand and to give feedback along the way.

When you are engaged in *defensive communication*, you are afraid the other person is trying to change you. You tend to not listen, instead stockpiling ammunition for later. You think you cannot listen to the other person because you will have to change, will feel guilty, or will be blamed or shamed. You listen just enough to gather information to win the argument. Somewhere between *collaborative listening* (listening with your heart) and *defensive listening* (which is not listening), there is listening with your ears. While this is a common experience, it is not as fulfilling as listening with your heart.

There is also *collaborative speaking*, which involves sharing with the other person. In this case, you want to share your truth so the person listening can see the real you. You speak in a way that allows the recipient to drop defenses and really hear what you are saying. In this mode, you would use a lot of *process language*, such as verbs that describe what you see, feel, and think in present time. You use *'I' statements*, indicating your willingness to have the other person know you better. These are statements that start with the pronoun *I*, meaning that you are talking about yourself and your own experience. With this communication style, you risk being vulnerable, but it is usually a risk worth taking. *'You' statements*, on the other hand, tend to describe the other person accusingly or in an unflattering way and result in raised defenses.

Defensive speaking involves talking at the other person.[21] You tell the individual information so that he or she will change. You use a lot of *static language* such as nouns and labels, and you speak in a way that is blaming, accusing, and guilt-inducing. You tend to think that things are the other person's fault. You think your truth is the only truth and try to make the other person seem wrong. Refrains repeated either in your mind or aloud start with, "You're always," "Why can't you," "You never," and "Remember when you." The tone is often blaming, shaming, guilting, teasing, or sarcastic. It's not one that evokes good feelings!

When you have conflict with someone in your life, or even just difficulty communicating with each other, it is helpful to clarify what the other person is saying. We each start with an agenda or something we want to see happen. It is helpful to hear the other person's full agenda before rebutting statements, asking questions, or starting on your own agenda. As we noted earlier, it's a good idea to refrain from interrupting unless you truly need to have the person clarify something.

After the other person has spoken, it is helpful to use the "I heard you say" (IHUS) paradigm, and then give the person the chance to clarify again.[22] This process is also known as paraphrasing the other person's words. It allows you to understand the speaker as fully as possible, and it gives the speaker a chance to augment or refine his or her statements. This is not a time to disagree or argue, but only to take in what the other person is saying without judgment. This creates safety in the communication process. Once you start employing it, you may be surprised to find how often you had an internal agenda or an expectation concerning what you thought the other person was going to say—and how surprised you are by the unexpected information you received.

Nonviolent Communication, a book by Marshall B. Rosenberg, includes a section called "Building a Vocabulary for Feelings" (see appendix 3).[23] This section lists a number of adjectives that can be used to describe your feelings about life in a vivid way. Adjectives you might choose when you feel that your needs are being met include *alive, expansive,* and *peaceful*. Adjectives you might choose when you feel your needs are not being met include *angry, impatient,* and *withdrawn*. These adjectives are helpful to read and incorporate so that you can identify and articulate what you are feeling. Important in Rosenberg's work is his differentiation between "feeling words" and words that identify how we think others react or behave toward us.

An example might be that you would say, "I feel criticized." This response would be more that you think you are being criticized, given that 'criticized' is not a feeling. You may feel angry or hurt, and it may be connected to other times you have heard similar words when you were being criticized. In the moment, you may or may not have been experiencing criticism. Nevertheless, it is not a feeling. When communicating, it is important to differentiate between your feelings and your thoughts.

Rosenberg has developed what he calls the NVC (Nonviolent Communication) Process, which is very valuable for collaborative communication. Its four components are *observations, feelings, needs,* and *requests*.

According to Rosenberg, the list below defines the elements that we need to be prepared to communicate:

1. The concrete actions we *observe* that affect our well-being.
2. How we *feel* in relation to what we observe.
3. The *needs*, values, desire, etc. that create our feelings.
4. The concrete actions we *request* in order to enrich our lives.[24]

An example of this positive communication might be a husband making the following statements to his wife: "I see that you have made several purchases that didn't get listed in the checkbook. When you do this, I feel frustrated and get confused trying to balance the checkbook. What I need is to stay organized so I can manage our budget better. My request is that you either write the purchases down, or even call home and leave a message on the recorder listing the place of the purchase and the amount."

This is very different from the communication below:

"I am really let down that you messed up the checkbook again. This messes everything up and takes me hours to fix. Why can't you just take the time to do it right? I already feel overworked and now there is this mess to fix."

Can you see how the first example is one in which the wife would be more apt to listen and want to change her behavior? In the second example, she may respond by blaming, arguing, denying, or withdrawing. You may want to notice your own communication styles and ask yourself, "Am I communicating in a way that allows the other person to truly hear and understand me?" Use the above information to adjust your communication as needed.

Tools and Exercises

1. Practice changing your thoughts and feelings when you are in a public situation and find yourself reacting with anger or another feeling that you would prefer not to feel. Afterward, write about your experience in your journal. This is like other practices. At first it may seem difficult, but after you have tried the technique several times, you realize that what happened was not important in the larger picture of life, happiness, and health.

2. Pay attention to the things on which you are focusing. Start when you first awake. Where does your mind go? What thoughts come through? At this time, you are just noticing, but it will be helpful to have a positive image or short statement for yourself to replace any negativity. You may just say something simple like, "I choose happiness in this moment," or "I forgive myself for what I have or have not done."

3. How do you change your thoughts and feelings? The first step is to get in touch with your self-talk. You chatter to yourself all day long, but you probably don't notice. Slow down and begin to listen to your thoughts. One way to do this is to

write them down. Notice your thoughts throughout the day and just write them down. You might try setting a timer to go off at regular intervals throughout the day to remind you to note your thoughts. Do this for a few days. After these few days have passed, continue to write down your thoughts, but then also challenge them.

For example, a man wants to apply for a new position in his company. As he anticipates the interview he thinks, "I won't get the job; they will want someone else, not me." He writes this down and then challenges it.

Thought: I won't get the job. They will want someone else, not me.

Challenge: Wait a minute. You don't know who they will want. You are not in their heads. You have all the skills they need and more. You have worked for this company for five years and continue to make them a lot of money. You are on time, and you do not create problems. You would be a great choice for this new position. If you do not get it, it is because there is a better position for you in the future.

Now, had the interviewee not written this down, he might not have realized he was criticizing himself. He also would not have accessed the part of himself that is there to self-support. Once you access this part of yourself, it becomes louder and louder! It is wonderful to learn to look within for the love and support you so often look for outside of yourself.

4. In my meditation classes, I teach the tool of being in the center of the head.[25] Imagine a situation in which you normally find yourself reacting or feeling someone else's feelings. Then close your eyes and bring your attention the center of your head. This is the place behind and above your eyes and between your ears. This is a place of neutrality, a place where you can look out and see as if you were looking at a movie screen. You are not pushing anything away or pulling anything toward you. The center of the head is where you see things with neutrality and amusement. Notice how separate you feel from the other people's emotions in this state.

5. Identify the way or ways in which you express anger. Do you have outbursts at others? Are you passive-aggressive in getting revenge or punishing others? Do you turn anger inward, withdrawing and becoming self-destructive? Take a few minutes to write about the last few times you were angry to help evaluate your anger response honestly.

6. Read through the section on boundaries and make a self-assessment. Identify your own collapsed boundaries, rigid boundaries, and healthy boundaries. Use the journal process to go deeper into the experiences that created your protective responses.

7. Practice using the words in Building a Vocabulary for Feelings found in appendix 3.

8. We often have issues with others that remain present. You can use your journal to write a letter to those with whom you are angry or feel a need to communicate clearly, or you may choose to do a twenty-minute timed writing on the issue. Afterward, write out how you would communicate with this person using the NVC process.[26]

Week Eight: Prayer and Meditation

Prayer

Ministry is a service, and prior to the advent of large, organized religions such as Christianity, the person the community came to for counsel, healing, forgiveness, and ritual became what we call the minister. This organic process describes how my ministry initially came about. My undergraduate work at Gonzaga University was in psychology and religious studies. In graduate school at Gonzaga, I studied counseling psychology.

At that time, I also explored women's spirituality and learned how women circled together to share and heal. I had wanted to be a priest, but because I was a woman, this was not possible—at least in the Catholic Church. I loved the ritual of the Catholic Church, and as a convert, I had none of the shadow side of the church behind me. Having had my children when I was young, I was about twelve to fifteen years older than most of my classmates. I became good friends with a couple of women in class, and it happened that we got together for prayer and ritual on the weekends. I set a room up in my home for this purpose. They came to me to learn about connecting with the feminine side of God (the Goddess), and we attended Mass as well. At that time, it appeared to me that Jesus came to teach values that are traditionally seen as feminine, which is a distinct change from those presented in the Old Testament.

After we graduated, my friends moved back to the west side of Washington and entered doctoral programs in psychology. A few years after we graduated, one of these friends came back to Spokane for the weekend. She had a baby girl and asked me to baptize her. While I had no formal training as a minister, it felt right to her and her husband, as well as to me. This opened me up to understanding my role in life as a minister.

Not long after, my mother died quickly from cancer. She was diagnosed and then passed within two weeks. My brother and I arranged for the funeral, and as I had not been attending Mass for a while, I did not know the priest who came to preside over the funeral. Although he was a wonderful priest, he didn't know the family, and his eulogy lacked life and warmth. When I got up to speak about my mom, I felt an incredible energy come from above my head down my spine, and I felt an awe-inspiring and powerful presence. I talked about my mom and death, really feeling as if I had done it before. The supervisor from my job at the time—a tremendous woman whom I loved and who taught me so much—came to me afterward and said she had seen what happened. She said, "You were really in your element." Having her witness this experience was valuable to me. I understood that, yes, this was a part of who I am. I am a minister.

I became ordained a couple of years later in a ceremony with my dearest friend. She and I now have a small, non-traditional congregation. We are ordained in the International Association of Spiritual Healers and Earth Stewards (**http://www. shes.org**).[1] As I think about prayer, I realize that it has become so natural for me. Almost a constant behavior, it seems difficult to separate from my other thinking as I write about ways to pray.

When you have experienced pain or illness for a long period, I would imagine you have already prayed often. In exploring how important prayer is, let's examine and revisit the way in which you pray.

A verse in the New Testament assures us, "You will receive all that you pray for, provided you have faith" (Matthew 21:22). The way your parents and grandparents prayed may be different from how you pray today. Dr. Larry Dossey writes extensively about the power of prayer and healing in his 1993 book, *Healing Words*.[2] In it, he cites a study by Herbert Benson of Harvard University Medical School.

Working with his fellow researcher and physiologist, Robert Keith Wallace, Benson showed that when subjects meditated with a mantra that consisted of an Asian word containing no meaning for the meditator, with use it became charged with ritualistic value, and healthful body changes occurred. These included lower blood pressure, slower heart rate, and lower metabolic rates. Benson believed there was no magic in the mantra.

To test this suspicion, he taught people to meditate using the word *one* or any other phrase they found comfortable. He then studied Christians and Jews who prayed regularly. He asked Catholics to use mantra phrases such as "Hail Mary, full of grace," or "Lord Jesus Christ, have mercy upon me." Jews mainly used either the peace greeting of *shalom* or *echad*, which means "one." Protestants frequently chose the first line of the Lord's Prayer, "Our Father who art in heaven," or "The Lord is my shepherd," which is the opening of the Twenty-third Psalm. All of the mantras worked, and all were equally effective in stimulating the healthful physiological changes in the body that Benson called the "relaxation response." But Benson also found that those who used the word *one*, or similar simple phrases, didn't stick with the program. Conversely, those who used prayers rather than meaningless phrases continued.[3]

What this study shows me is that prayer, when used in this manner, is similar to meditation. One way to pray is to be repetitive. If you have ever used prayer beads or the rosary, you know this. Recital is another form of prayer. Many people use scripture from their religion as prayer. They may do this repetitively, or they may read scripture and then reflect on what it means. Others talk to God or their Higher Power as they would to a friend. I have often heard it said that prayer is talking to God, and meditation is listening.

One of my favorite ways of praying is to be in a walking meditation or walking prayer. Quiet and present, I walk along the river. I sense God all around me and often communicate with God. I connect well with nature and often sense the answers to my questions through it.

Journaling is another way to connect with the Divine. "Dear God" letters are often effective in clarifying where you have become stuck. Having a heart full of gratitude is another way of praying. When you expand your view of prayer this way, you may find that you pray often through the day. I am a believer in the notion that whatever we focus on becomes greater and grander in our lives, so take some time to focus on gratitude and love. See how this affects your pain.

Prayer and the need for prayer can be humorous and tragic. Several years ago, I remember standing in the hallway of my house between the bedroom and the living room. I was in a lot of pain and had been for many months. Stressed from overworking, I suffered from depression as well. I remember saying to God in an angry and insistent voice (I don't remember whether it was out loud or in my head), "Okay, God! If I have to be in a body, I'm going to have *fun*!" I was extremely distraught at this time, and as soon as I made my declaration, I heard the angels all around me laughing. I was shocked and surprised, but I understood. Much of my suffering was due to the fact that I was suffering. Having fun, playing, being light, and letting go was the answer to my prayer. It worked!

On a more serious note, I remember when I was working at a halfway house for young men who were transitioning from juvenile detention back into the community. I worked the swing shift, and at about seven o'clock in the evening, I got a call from my older daughter, Charisma. At the time, she was thirteen years old. My younger daughter, Misty, was twelve. "Mom, the house is on fire!" Charisma exclaimed. I told her to get herself and her sister out of the house immediately, and I would call the fire department and Grandpa.

As frightened as I was, I had to wait for another staff member to come and relieve me, and I prayed the entire time. When I left the facility, I prayed (screamed) at the top of my lungs, "Please God, protect my children! Please, Jesus! Please!" I drove home, and as I turned the corner, I saw my street filled with people. A fire truck and ambulance were there. Next to the ambulance I saw my dad, and next to him my children—watching the house burn. So grateful that my children were safe, I took my first deep breath, began to cry, and then I parked my car and joined my family. As I looked at the roof burning, I immediately saw the hand of Jesus reaching down into the house through the roof and bringing out Life. I sensed that this tragedy would bring new life and something good to my family. As it turned out, although I had lost almost everything, my home was gutted and rebuilt and became a beautiful new home. Of course, the main thing was that my children were safe. This was definitely a prayer answered.

Meditation

Before I share with you about meditation, I want to acknowledge that you may experience resistance to meditation at first. You may be fearful to sit and really experience what you are thinking or feeling, or you may not want to become aware of the sensations in your body. Even this morning as I awoke, I quickly shifted my thoughts from meditation to something else. Why did I do that? Why was I so afraid to listen to what my mind was saying? Usually I awake with new ideas and plans and creative ventures. This morning I didn't want to hear what I was thinking. I went back to catch the thought, and it was gone. When I sat up to read on my Kindle, I felt good. I looked at the calendar in my iPhone, and my day was set to write. It was a good day. What was I afraid to think about? I am sure it will surface in my meditation.

You may have this same experience. You may think there is just too much information in your mind, and you would never be able to quiet yourself, but it's really not so difficult. Take a moment and just sit with your eyes open. Look at what is in front of you. Look at whatever you see and focus on the detail. Experience your senses. Feel the chair under you. Notice how your breath changes. You are becoming more aware, more awake, more alive, and you are beginning to come to a meditative state. Another way to do this is to close your eyes and listen. Listen to the sounds that are far away. Now listen to the sounds that are close by. Allow yourself to become more aware and more meditative!

There are several ways to meditate. I have practiced walking meditation for over twenty years, in which I walk a loop along the Spokane River ... first along the river, then crossing over the bridge, walking the other side, and then crossing back. (It's hard not to love bridges on a meditative walk!) In this meditation, I am aware of all my senses. My mind is quiet. I can feel the energy of the trees and bushes as I walk by, as well as the earth under my feet. I can hear the sound of the river and feel the energy of the negative ions, bathing me with love. Negative ions are found in moving water and in sunny conditions. This is one reason people gravitate toward moving rivers, waterfalls, and oceans. According to Michael Terman of Columbia University Medical Center, "Negative ions are naturally occurring charged air particles that are always circulating in the environment around you." He says that summer air is highly concentrated with the negative ions, and high negative ions evoke "beneficial mood effects." (**http://asp.cumc.columbia.edu/psych/asktheexperts/ask_th e_experts_inquiry .asp?SI=102**).

Occasionally in this walk, I receive a specific piece of information, such as the time I understood a tree I often walked by had "grandmother energy." After that, I called her the grandmother tree. When I was in need of wisdom, I would ask my question before I began the walk and allowed the grandmother tree to guide me. I also understood a certain place on the path along the river was "womb energy." This energy was about creation, and there I received information regarding what I wanted to birth next.

In the 1990s, from the Church of Divine Man, I learned and practiced a guided meditation that included steps such as grounding, centering, and running my earth and cosmic energy. After having a few psychic readings from members of this church, I was automatically able to read myself and others.

What was most difficult for me was learning to have a sitting meditation where I quieted my mind. In subsequently learning to practice a sitting meditation, I noticed a couple of things. One is that it took me a long time to learn to meditate this way. I went to a friend of mine who is a psychiatrist and a shaman, visiting with him each Saturday morning for months. I kept saying, "I know I need to meditate, but I just can't do it." He and I would meditate together, but I still just couldn't manage to do it on my own. He would teach me, we would practice, and I would resist. I was trying to meditate after work, around five or six o'clock. I would sit down, and my mind would be full of junk thoughts. It would swirl with information, which was actually tiring for me. I was tiring because of my resistance.

I eventually decided to meditate first thing in the morning, and this changed my experience exponentially. I awoke, sat up straight, connected my thumb, index, and middle finger on my knees or in my lap, depending upon where Mattie Grace (my large, grey, polydactyl cat) had settled, and the experience was wonderful. While some images from dreams and certain thoughts about what I needed to do for the day would pass through, most of the time I just drifted into that peaceful place and enjoyed the experience.

At first I set my timer for twenty minutes, and it was admittedly difficult to meditate that long, so I would take a deep breath and go in for another round. Soon though, the twenty-minute timer interrupted my experience. After that, while I did glance at my clock before I meditated, I no longer used a timer. I could go as long as I desired and realized my pattern was to meditate, come up a little, then take a deep breath and go back down. I can still do this over as long a period of time as I would like, allowing the meditation to carry me.

I'll share more later about the great teachings and experiences that I have learned through my meditation, but first I want to talk to you about the general practice itself.

Meditation is an ancient practice, and there are numerous types and methods. I am not an expert at meditation, but I am happy to share my experience and knowledge on the subject with you. Today, many people use meditation to help with stress, calm themselves, and explore beyond their conscious minds. In this book, I outline a few ways to meditate in order to expand your awareness, as well as later introducing guided imagery to help with healing.

You may want to use meditation as a positive choice in managing your mood. It can be used as an alternative or an addition to medication. As seen in the earlier example of Alice in Week One, as you change your thinking, your feelings change as well.

Some meditation methods ask you to sit quietly and clear your mind, while other methods have you focus your awareness. This can be achieved by focusing on various things such as your breathing, a particular part of your body, the space above your head, or in following a specific visualization.

My first experience with meditation was with Transcendental Meditation (TM) in the 1970s. Transcendental Meditation began in India with Maharishi Mahesh Yogi in the 1950s and expanded to other countries, becoming even more popular by the time I began to learn the practice. I don't really remember how I ended up in this meditation group, and I didn't practice this type of meditation for long, so I won't expound on it here. There are many resources on what is known as TM.

Instead, I learned the meditation I have practiced most in my life at the Church of Divine Man—guided meditation. Mary Ellen Flora, the church founder, writes in her book, *Meditation: Key to Spiritual Awakening*:

> The purpose of meditation is to communicate with the Cosmic Consciousness or God. This ultimate purpose of meditation, to re-establish your one-to-one communication with God, takes you on a journey of getting to know yourself and your creations. As you turn within during meditation, you find your path to God within you. You learn to see yourself as the creator of your reality and the one who decides your fate. You realize that each lifetime offers learning opportunities, and meditation can help you use each life to the fullest. If you do not focus on your spiritual lesson, you return repeatedly in other lives until you learn that lesson.[4]

My favorite explanation of the benefits of meditation comes from Deepak Chopra's *Quantum Healing: Exploring the Frontiers of Mind/Body Medicine*, which I talked about when addressing feelings in Week Five.[5] Chopra describes our consciousness as being similar to the strings on a violin. The violin has one pitch, but the pitch changes as your fingers move along the string. This is similar to your body and health changing with your "subjective moods, fleeting desires, and swings of emotion." Chopra notes that for most people the pitch is consistent. He uses the example of how "a depressed person radiates depression even when he forces himself to act positive," and "a hostile person can set a whole room on edge, even when he says the most harmless things."[6] He explains that although there is a variation in moods, a person's behavior is determined by his or her usual pitch, and people cannot think themselves to a higher vibration. However, they can slide into a new pitch using meditation, thereby expanding their minds beyond the usual limitations. Meditation allows the mind to move beyond itself by transcending the fixed level through silence and being devoid of thoughts.

One value of meditating with a friend is that we can match each other's energy and vibration. Remember back to the shaman I mentioned earlier; this psychiatrist/shaman is my dear friend. I called him again when I found myself stuck and sluggish while writing this book. We met for a movie and dinner, and afterwards I asked him if we could meditate together. I knew that he had accessed a level of meditation beyond that which I could attain. I told him I wanted to clear up some behaviors and raise my vibration. As we sat together with our eyes closed, he instructed me to follow him. We sat silently for an unknown length of time, during which I found myself following him upward through colors and shapes. I reached a breakthrough to a height I had not reached before, and immediately afterward I was able to access a part of myself I had not yet experienced. When evaluating situations, I am able to access the higher part of myself, my Higher Self, to see clearly the difference between my Higher Self and my Ego. This is the result of one meditative experience with someone who has attained what he calls *emptiness*.

Every religious community has its own way of praying and meditating. While it's important for you to find the process most comfortable for you, it is likely more important to find the one you will actually practice on a regular basis. Below, you will find that I have sorted the meditations into three types: concentration, mindfulness, and guided imagery.

Concentration Meditation

When practicing concentration meditation, you focus your attention on your breath, an image, or a sound (mantra) in order to still your mind and allow a greater awareness and clarity to emerge. This is similar to zooming in and narrowing the focus to a particular object or field

Breathing Meditation

The most common meditation practice is focusing on your breath. Through this continued focus, the "mind clutter" begins to quiet, and you gain a sense of calmness and relaxation. Over time and with practice, the thoughts that were once racing or popping into your mind calm down, and a sense of peace takes over. As you focus on the breath, the rhythmic inhalation and exhalation deepens the breathing, and your mind and body become tranquil.

The simplest form of breathing meditation is to just focus on your breath. Obviously, breath is an integral part of your existence. Begin by focusing on your breathing, noticing it moving in and out of your nostrils. You could also focus on your chest and notice as it gently moves up and down.

I like to focus on my belly and feel how it expands as I breathe in, as well as how it contracts as I breathe out. This is called diaphragmatic breathing and is less likely to cause hyperventilation than breathing into the chest, which is considered shallow breathing. It is a good place to start for beginning meditators. When you focus on your breath, be sure to just notice and not think about how you are doing it. Be passive to the process. It is an experience you will learn from, not one that you have to learn. The practice of focusing on your breath will relax you and can be the beginning of your journey.

A more intense practice of focusing on the breath is pranayama breathing, which is a yogic practice. According to Swami Sivananda Rhada, this is a process of breath control. The purpose of this type of meditation is to connect with the cosmos and gain control over your central nervous system and mind.[7] It is best practiced with character building and to learn to manage the lower physical self. This is a practice of alternate nostril breathing. "Character building" and "managing your lower physical self" means taking control over your thoughts and behaviors that no longer serve you, while creating new, positive, healthy thoughts and behaviors.

I first became aware of pranayama breathing when I traveled to India with a friend of mine who has a home in India but currently lives in the United States. He said that his uncle taught him this practice. When we were at his home in Kolkata (formerly Calcutta), he sat cross-legged on the floor every morning and practiced this breathing for twenty to thirty minutes. This practice increases the alpha waves, and the benefits if executed correctly are to calm the mind, gain control over the emotions, refine the senses, and remove all selfish desires while gaining a sense of peace and harmony. It has also been said to balance the right and left brain.

Various teachers may instruct you to do this differently, but a simple method follows:

1. Close the right nostril with your right thumb, and inhale through the left nostril to the count of four seconds.

2. Then close the left nostril with your right ring finger and little finger. At the same time, remove your thumb from the right nostril. Exhale through this nostril to the count of eight seconds.

3. Next, inhale through the right nostril to the count of four seconds. Close your right nostril with your right thumb, and exhale through the left nostril to the count of eight seconds.

4. This is one round. It is recommended to start slowly with a few rounds and build up.

Swami Radha shares extensive information on this practice with different counts than what I outlined for you above. She says relaxation is essential to the practice and offers some preliminary neck and shoulder exercises to develop. She notes the benefits as release of karma and destruction of illusion, proper elimination of carbon dioxide and absorption of oxygen, as well as calmness, control over the mind, a sense of peace and harmony, an increased ability to observe, and a relaxation for your heart and nervous system.

Focusing on an Object

Focusing on an object is another choice for concentration meditation. There are several objects you can use, but I suggest you find one that is pleasing to you. You could focus on an external object such as a candle flame, a bowl, a flower, or a photo of someone you love. You could also choose a photo of Jesus, Buddha, or an angel. Another method is to focus in the center of your head—the space above and behind your eyes, in the middle of your head. This is a place of neutrality as taught by the Church of Divine Man.[8] You may instead choose to focus either between your eyes or in the center of your heart. Another common place to practice focus is in your belly, three fingers below your belly button and inside a few inches. The conscious focus in the above examples is on the candle, photo, or particular body part. However, in focusing on those literal objects, you become aware of the breathing as well, and you experience a calm, relaxed, tranquil state of being.

Using a Mantra

A third concentration meditation involves using a mantra. A mantra, as previously described, is a short phrase with an easy rhythm used to increase results. A mantra is used to suggest a favorable state of being. To reiterate from earlier in this book, a good early morning mantra is, "I am alive, awake, refreshed, and protected from stress." My favorite walking mantra is, "I am strong, healthy, and fit." Mantras originated in the Vedic tradition of enlightenment in India and have since been incorporated by many traditions.

According to "The Power of Mantra Chanting," an article by Gyan Rajhans, "The sacred utterances or chanting of Sanskrit Mantras provide us with the power to attain our goals and lift ourselves from the ordinary to the higher level of consciousness."[9] This is believed to be so because "different sounds have different effects on the human psyche."[10]

Hindus believe that Sanskrit mantras are the most powerful, but I find English mantras to be powerful as well. When using mantras, you may chant a repetition of the same words or sounds repeatedly, using the chant as sound or as vibration. Mantras range from simple words to complex sounds with specific pitches and ranges. The ancient chants of India may have marked the beginning of this type of healing.

According to the article entitled "Mantras and Sacred Symbols," many believe that "there are mantras that accomplish many kinds of wondrous deeds simply by correctly chanting them," and that "other mantras help purify one's consciousness, give spiritual enlightenment, and put one in touch with the Supreme."[11] Repeating a mantra is a spiritual technique that calms the mind and makes one more attuned to Spirit.

Mindfulness Meditation

The practice of mindfulness meditation comes from Buddhism and has been taught by many in the West. In mindfulness meditation, you focus on the present moment and not the past or the future. While you notice your thoughts, you realize that they are just thoughts and let them go by. This is done with awareness that that your thoughts are simply your thoughts, and that you are not your thoughts. This meditation can be done at any time. It is a daily practice of awareness in the present moment. This is the practice previously mentioned that happened naturally for me as I took my daily walk along the Spokane River. If you remember, I noticed the bottom of my feet connecting with the earth at each step. I became more aware of and present to each bird that passed, as well as the many leaves and rocks through which I walked. Every day, I walked by a particular tree, and I began to sense it as having the energy of a grandmother.

The value of therapeutic healing that comes from meditation has been well researched. Dr. Jon Kabat-Zinn has written extensively about this topic and developed a program called Mindfulness-Based Stress Reduction (MBSR).[12] This program is used as a complementary form of medicine in over 200 hospitals in the United States. Kabat-Zinn is a professor of medicine, emeritus and founding director of the Stress Reduction Clinic and the Center for Mindfulness in Medicine, Health Care, and Society at the University of Massachusetts Medical School. He teaches mindfulness meditation as a technique to help people cope with stress, anxiety, pain, and illness. Other research shows that mindfulness can increase functioning in those who experience chronic pain.[13] Mindfulness increases day-to-day awareness.

There are many ways to practice mindfulness meditation. One that I particularly enjoy is to focus on the sounds close by and then the sounds that are far away. This takes me into a state of meditation that I enjoy, which is just being present.

Another way to practice mindfulness meditation is through a body scan, which I have learned in several classes. Most recently, I've been using it for trauma healing, in conjunction with EMDR. You can start at the top of your head and just let your attention slowly move down your head, then down the trunk of your body, followed by your arms, and then your lower body ... one leg and one foot at a time. Notice any sensations you feel and be present to those feelings. The sensations may change as you do this; just let it happen. When I practice the body scan, I often get intuitive information about my body, but that is not the purpose of it. Just allow yourself to be present. Afterward, you can write anything you wish about the experience in your journal.

Guided Meditation

Guided meditation is similar to hypnotherapy. In guided meditation, a person or a recorded script guides you into a meditative state. You can also take yourself through guided imagery with a script or with awareness of the images you would like to create.

As with hypnotherapy, guided imagery uses all of your senses, yet guided imagery is different in that it focuses and directs your imagination. When the mind is imagining, the body responds as if what it sees is true. An example of this might include imagining a vacation. Let's pick a beach resort. As you are sitting at your desk at work, you find yourself drifting to the beach, feeling the sun on your face, smelling the sea, and imaging the taste of a fresh, cold lemonade next to you. Your body may relax as your breathing slows down and time speeds up. This is an example of going into trance and experiencing whatever you imagine.

I experienced this phenomenon myself in a much different way when I went to see the movie remake of *A War of the Worlds*. As I sat close to the big screen, I couldn't help but cover my face to protect myself from the intensity of the alien moving through the city. Was I really in danger? No, but my body certainly responded with adrenaline as if I were.

Guided imagery is used for many purposes, and the imagery selected will depend on your goal. For instance, if you want to manage your pain, the imagery may be full of metaphors that help you to connect with your subconscious mind. For example, when I awake in the morning with pain in my neck from sleeping, during meditation I image a blue light coming down from the top of my head into the painful areas of my neck and shoulders. As I do this, I see the blue light cooling off the inflammation in my neck and shoulders. Within a minute or so, the pain is gone. (Remember that I have been practicing for quite some time, and this technique is a result of the practice. Do not be discouraged if you try this and it does not work for you immediately.) For another example, if you want to stop smoking, the images may be of practicing new behaviors, such as picking up the crossword puzzle book when your hands are used to picking up a cigarette.

Guided imagery is also helpful in creating feelings of safety or empowerment. Sometimes when I am working with a client, images of past traumas surface, and I often use imagery to help the client feel safe and reorient him or her to present time before the session ends. If you are interested in learning a guided meditation that teaches you self-healing tools and takes you through a process of clearing your chakras, you can use my CD, *Chakra Clearing*.[14]

Now I will share with you one of the incredible experiences that has come to me in meditation. I may even write a book about this process once it is completely understood. In meditation recently I saw the symbol of a bright golden spiral in my heart. My inner meditation guide instructed me to spin this spiral, and so I did. The spiral spun a golden light throughout my body and out to about 12 inches *surrounding* my body. I immediately felt warmth, love, and protection. I understood this was the way for me to protect my energetic field and prepare for meditation after I grounded myself.

There are additional parts to this that have been given to me, and I will understand them more as I meditate. One was the symbol of a beautiful diamond that was at my brow chakra between my eyes. The third symbol given to me was that of a flaming circle at the 8th chakra, which is above the crown chakra. I understand this chakra to hold the akashic records, which are said to contain all records of humans and the Universe. At this time, more information is being given about this symbol, which I will share in another writing. Throughout my life, I have received information that makes sense and doesn't make sense, but I have written and continue to write what I get in my journals, and I trust the process. I hope you will do this as well.

Make no mistake, whether prayer or meditation, the process stills the chatter and voices within so you can hear your own inner guidance—the voice of God/Goddess or your Guides. Prayer and meditation allow you to open yourself to wisdom and healing beyond what your Ego dictates or allows.

Through the practice of prayer and meditation, Spirit comes through and enters your heart! In the Christian faith, this is referred to this as the Holy Spirit. I am sure other religions each have their own word for it, but researching and outlining those terms is not within the scope of this particular book. I welcome your interest in researching them yourself, and I recommend that you do so if you feel moved in that direction.

No matter what you call it, when you achieve inner peace, the world around you feels peaceful.

Tools and Exercises

Ways to Pray

Think about some of the ways in which you pray. Use the examples below to explore new methods.

1. Write out your prayers in your journal. Write about what you would like the Divine to help you with, what you would like to create, and what you would like the Divine to know. Ask for prayers for others in your journal. Write down twenty things you are grateful for, then go back in a month or so and reread your journal entry. You may be amazed at prayers answered.

2. Use scripture or writings that are important to you for prayer. You can memorize these words and recite them, or you can read a passage (silently or aloud) and reflect. Ask for guidance as you focus on these words.

3. Start a walking prayer practice. Walk in nature and feel your heart grow full of gratitude at the sun or snow, flowers, trees, squirrels, or whatever nature you find. You can also walk in your neighborhood and thank God or pray for your neighbors.

4. Pray for others. Quiet yourself and just let people and situations come to mind, and ask for the Highest Good for this person or this situation.

5. Sit and focus in your heart, and feel gratitude. Think about something that brings you joy, and then increase this feeling of gratitude, imagining it emanating from you to the hearts of others—both individuals and groups. Surround your block, city, state, country, and planet with this incredible love from your heart.

Ways to Meditate

Enjoy a walking meditation. Take a walk where you will not be significantly distracted by cars or others. Walk with a presence of being in the moment. Focus on your breathing, or feel the bottom of your feet on the ground. Become aware of all your senses.

1. Practice concentration meditation using your breath. You can use the practice I described, or you can just focus on your breathing. Take notes afterward in your journal.

2. Practice concentration meditation using an image or an object. Allow your mind to continue to return to the image or object. Take notes afterward in your journal.

3. Practice concentration meditation using a mantra. You may want to create your own mantra or take one from the Bible or a text. Take notes afterward in your journal.

4. Practice mindfulness meditation. Bring your awareness into present time and just let thoughts

pass. Don't pull them toward you or push them away. Just stay present. Take notes afterward in your journal.

5. Use a guided meditation CD in order to experience guided meditation. Take notes afterward in your journal.

Week Nine: Trauma

This week we will focus on healing trauma. Although most of us think about trauma in terms of combat situations or something tantamount to seeing a murder on the street, nearly all people have experienced some kind of trauma. Whether you remember the original trauma or not, you still have the symptoms. Different individuals respond differently to situations, so one person can become traumatized by a specific instance while another is not.

In 1997, Peter Levine and Ann Frederick wrote a book called *Waking the Tiger: Healing Trauma: The Innate Capacity to Transform Overwhelming Experiences.*[1] You may be surprised to hear it, but the authors affirm, "Trauma has become so commonplace that most people don't even recognize its presence." Levine and Frederick list some events that people have experienced which resulted in traumatic reactions later in their life, including fetal trauma (intra-uterine), birth trauma, loss of a parent or close family member, illness, physical injury, sexual or emotional abuse, witnessing violence, tonsillectomies with ether, being present in natural disasters, dental procedures, surgery, and more.[2]

It is interesting that so many traumas come from routine medical procedures. I remember one of my own several years ago for the removal of a lump in my breast. I had already been traumatized by the hospital experience after my head injury at age fourteen. Looking back, I see the trauma of the hospital experience when I was fourteen years old as having stayed with me. In a state of protective denial, I underwent the surgical procedure for my breast, despite intuition clearly telling me the lump was benign. Because of this decision, I felt as if I was on the medical industry's conveyor belt. So, when the nurse made the appointment for the surgery, I went along with it. I was fortunate that a good friend of mine accompanied me to the hospital. Before surgery, she took me through a guided meditation in which she described little angel hands gently and carefully going in and loosening and removing the lump. The experience was gentle and comforting; it replaced my previous negative, fearful, and traumatic images with positive ones.

Posttraumatic Stress Disorder

There is a high correlation between physical pain and posttraumatic stress disorder (PTSD). You may even be suffering from PTSD without knowing it. As I describe the symptoms, take some time to assess yourself and whether or not the symptoms match your own experience. The DSM-IV-TR, the American Psychiatric Association's manual of disorders, explains that a diagnosis of PTSD is likely when a person has "experienced, witnessed, or was confronted with an event or events that involve actual or threatened death or serious injury, or a threat to the physical integrity of self or others," or that "the person's response involved intense fear, helplessness, or horror."[3]

Francine Shapiro, the author and originator of eye movement desensitization and reprocessing (EMDR), refers to trauma as being either *big T's* (big traumas) or *little t's* (little traumas).[4] For instance, when my house burned, it was definitely a *big T*. A memory of losing a pet when I was a child is a *little t*. Whether a situation is one or the other is subjective and dependent on the experience of each person.

When you think about traumas that may be underlying your pain, you may want to finish these statements in your mind or in your journal. I prefer the journal, and I will suggest again that if you truly want to experience the healing this book offers, *you will complete the process with the assistance of journaling.*

You may have reoccurring thoughts, images, or flashbacks to a situation. List them with regard to the following:

I have reoccurring thoughts about …

I can't stop having images of …

I keep dreaming about …

I go into a daze when I think about …

I often drink to forget …

I panic when I think of or remember …

I feel fear and anxiety when I remember …

My heart races when I remember …

I have a hard time breathing when I think about …

I am so sad when I remember …

You may also find yourself trying to avoid situations that have to do with the trauma. Complete these sentence stems:

I try to avoid thinking about …

I don't talk to people who remind me of …

I leave or feel numb when others bring up …

Whenever I can, I avoid going to (place) …

Whenever I can, I avoid (person) …

Whenever I can, I avoid (activity) …

I sense something happened when I was …

I can't remember exactly what happened, but I sense

…

People make me uncomfortable, because ...

People make me uncomfortable, since the time that ...

I don't feel much anymore, because ...

I don't feel much anymore, since the time that ...

I am not happy any longer, because ...

I am not happy any longer, since the time that ...

The future is no longer pleasant, because ...

The future is no longer pleasant, since the time that ...

Other symptoms may arise after a traumatic incident. Complete *these* sentence stems as well:

Sleep is difficult for me, since the time that ...

I feel so angry now that ...

I can't seem to concentrate since ...

I am so reactive to ...

I am startled more often now that ...

Symptoms of Trauma

When you experience trauma, your nervous system compensates for being in a continual state of high-level alertness by adapting. These adaptations then become symptoms. Initially, the physical symptoms of trauma can include a hyper-aroused state in which your heartbeat increases, your muscles tense, and you have difficulty breathing. Emotional symptoms of trauma can initially include shock, denial, and disbelief. Your system is not ready to process the information, and this denial is a helpful response.

The above responses happen immediately, while other symptoms begin to show up later and may last for years. Those symptoms may include the following:

- Hypervigilance (being on guard at all times)
- Anger, irritability, and mood swings
- Feelings of guilt, shame, or self-blame
- Feeling sad, hopeless, and helpless
- Confusion and difficulty concentrating
- Withdrawing from others and activities
- Feeling disconnected from others
- Feeling numb
- Intrusive images or flashbacks
- Extreme sensitivity to light and sound
- Hyperactivity
- Exaggerated emotional and startle responses
- Fatigue
- Aches and pains
- Muscle tension
- Difficulty sleeping
- Nightmares and night terrors

Let's look more closely at some of the symptoms of trauma. You may be aware of these in yourself or others, and you can see other symptoms listed in appendix 4: Symptoms of Trauma.

Hypervigilance

A definition of hypervigilance that I endorse can be found in the open source online encyclopedia, Wikipedia:

> Hypervigilance is an enhanced state of sensory sensitivity accompanied by an exaggerated intensity of behaviors whose purpose is to detect threats. Hypervigilance is also accompanied by a state of increased anxiety, which can cause exhaustion. Other symptoms include: abnormally increased arousal, a high responsiveness to stimuli and a constant scanning of the environment for threats.[5]

If you are hypervigilant, it may be that when you walk into a room you take in all aspects of it. You immediately assess who is there, where they are standing, whether they are familiar to you or not, and where the exits are. For the most part, you don't even realize you are doing all of this. Some people who have experienced trauma develop a stronger sixth sense, and this becomes a form of protection. Others become numb and are in denial of what is around them, which we will talk about later.

As I mentioned earlier, I grew up in a home with domestic violence and then received a head injury at age fourteen that nearly killed me. I remember my own experiences with hypervigilance. It was not until I was a chemical dependency counselor at an agency where we provided evaluations and urinalysis testing that I became aware of it. The director of the program was a woman who was extremely bright and loving, and she gave me a lot of feedback about myself. I learned about how my survival skills (hypervigilance and others) either added to my abilities as a chemical dependency counselor or got in the way. I know my own sixth sense increased a great deal, and my hypervigilance became connected to my intuition.

The agency for which I worked acted as a liaison between the criminal justice system and the chemical dependency treatment agencies; therefore, most of our clients were felons. One client—we'll call him Alan—was a sex offender. My office was toward the back of the building, down the hall, around the corner, and next to the director's office. The director was visiting with me in my office one day. I felt a little bit of fear come over me, and when I checked in with this feeling, I saw Alan in my mind. I looked at the director and said, "Alan just came in."

She looked at me and asked, "Really?"

When she went to check, she saw that I was right, and she had the chance to confirm it again another time after Alan came in. I stuck my head in her door, saying, "He's here."

I believe that most of us can do this when we learn to quiet and listen to ourselves, but those of us who have been traumatized often develop an extra sensitive ability. Again, this happens only if we do not choose to shut down that awareness to feel safe.

As we discussed earlier, you may not be aware of how these symptoms affect you until you are triggered by a current situation in which your "buttons get pushed" or you have a strong reaction to something that does not seem to merit that kind of emotional or physiological response. Whenever you have an exaggerated response to something in the current moment, it is attached to a memory (conscious or unconscious) from the past.

You may not be aware that the current pain you experience may be connected to a past traumatic experience. As stated earlier in this week, we tend to think of trauma in terms of what Francine Shapiro, originator of eye movement desensitization and reprocessing (EMDR), refers to as *big T's*—big traumas—that are perceived as life-threatening.[6] Such events include "combat, crimes such as rape, kidnapping, and assault; and natural disasters such as earthquakes, tornadoes, fires and floods."[7] However, Shapiro notes that damage also is done to our psyches by *little t's* that "occur in the innocuous but upsetting experiences that daily life sends our way."[8] These traumas may include losing a job, having to give up a class you wanted to take, or other experiences that affect your life significantly by generating important beliefs—they just may not be correlated in your mind with those beliefs.

Shapiro (1997) gives the example of Paul, who was her client in the early days of using EMDR. Paul had been

> diagnosed with AIDS and wanted to pursue some alternative methods of healing but found his efforts sabotaged by his belief, "I can't go after and get what I want." Paul had no memory to explain why he felt that way, but he remembered always believing it and felt it had held him back his whole life. He came in for help when he recognized his belief might prevent him from living his last days to the fullest.[9]

Shapiro described how she had Paul hold the belief in mind as she used the eye movements, and how he felt a strange sensation move down his arm. Shapiro had Paul focus on the belief and the sensation, and when he did so, he saw himself in his imagination as a four-year-old boy. He was playing at the top of the stairs with a ball. His mother told him not to go down the stairs, but when his ball fell, Paul went after it, tripping and falling on his arm. His mother went after him, pulled him by the arm, and spanked him. Paul recorded this in his mind as being punished for going after what he wanted. Having cleared this belief with Dr. Shapiro, he was then able to access the alternative health care he wanted and "embraced life with more freedom in his final years."[10]

This is just one example of the many successes achieved through this form of therapy. EMDR can be a very effective tool for processing forgotten traumas and clearing unhelpful beliefs. I offer you a better understanding of this later in the week.

Dissociation

Another sign of trauma you may experience is dissociation. The dissociation continuum can range from mild spaciness to dissociative identity disorder. When trauma happens and you dissociate, you may not remember the original trauma, but you will recognize symptoms that alert you to the existence of trauma in your past.

Some of the symptoms of dissociation are feelings of intense fear and helplessness, which may become chronic helplessness. You may continue to re-experience the traumatic event or have physical and emotional reactions to situations that are triggered by the original event, regardless of whether you have any conscious memory of it. You may also avoid situations—knowingly or not—that are associated with it. There may be a denial of the experience. There may be feelings of arousal or of numbing. You may experience traumatic anxiety and, in severe cases, hallucinations or paranoid ideation.

According to Levine and Frederick, a person experiences chronic helplessness when the "freezing, orienting, and defending responses become so fixated and weakened" that they move primarily along predetermined and dysfunctional pathways.[11] These responses, in conjunction with hypervigilance and an inability to learn new behaviors, leave the person helpless. Rather than continuing to move into new behaviors, the person withdraws into immobility. When the individual feels aroused, he or she moves directly into immobility. There may be an adrenaline response, but the person just freezes. This happens often in relationships. The person knows the relationship is not healthy, but is unable to move out of the relationship, even if there are other opportunities. The same dynamic applies to jobs.

Given my counseling experience, it would be remiss of me not to explore childhood sexual abuse at this point. Again, there is a high correlation between chronic pain and trauma. In my experience, there is also a high correlation between childhood sexual abuse and pain. I see a similar correlation between childhood sexual abuse and obesity.

In the nineties, the agency I worked for contracted me to provide chemical dependency counseling at Geiger Federal Prison in Spokane, Washington. I worked with many women there who had been convicted of drug possession. This was a time when our government enforced a conspiracy law, which meant that if you were aware of someone growing, manufacturing, or distributing drugs— but you didn't alert the authorities—you could be arrested, convicted, sentenced, and sent to prison. Many of the women I counseled were in relationships with men who were growing or selling marijuana. These women typically were convicted and sentenced to five years in a federal prison.

When I began counseling the clients, I focused on their relationships with the men in their lives and the difficulty that they had in being away from their children for so many years. Many of these women lived in California along the border of Mexico, and many were young mothers. In addition to the trauma of having been taken away from their children and families, they often had chemical dependency and codependency issues.

I believe it was after attending a workshop on women and sexual abuse that I became aware of the prevalence of sexual abuse in our society. When I returned to my office, I added the following question to the psychosocial questionnaire I used in the intake process: "Have you ever been sexually abused?" Previously, the question had not been asked, and sexual abuse had never been a treatment issue. After the question was added, nearly all of my clients—men and women alike—said that, as children, they had been sexually abused by adults! Common knowledge among many sexual abuse counselors is that in the United States, one in three girls and one in five boys are sexually abused.

My continued education in this area led me to a resource I highly recommend, which is a book by Ellen Bass and Laura Davis called *The Courage to Heal: A Guide for Women Survivors of Childhood Sexual Abuse.*[12] In appendix 5, I have included the Trauma Questionnaire, which is a list of questions I've developed that will help you make an assessment for yourself. If you find you have many of the symptoms, the book listed above can be extremely helpful in your healing. Again, I suggest you find a therapist trained in the treatment of sexual abuse to help you. One way to find a therapist is through your insurance company. Many agencies treat survivors of sexual abuse, and they should have a list of therapists in your area as well.

When I worked at Geiger Federal Prison, the nurses' station was just down the hall from my office. One day I had lunch with a nurse in the cafeteria. He was concerned about a mutual patient of ours with a rash. Developing a week before, the rash started at her chest and affected the entire trunk of her body. He had been giving her a topical ointment that wasn't helping. As soon as he said this, I saw an image of my client and how the healing had started inside her and was moving to the surface of her body. She and I had been focusing for the last few months on healing the childhood sexual abuse she had experienced, and she was nearly done with the issue. I could not share this information with the nurse, not only because I was bound by concerns for confidentiality, but also because I sensed he would not understand. When I talked to my client later that week, she shared that she knew the movement of the healing was causing the rash and agreed that she also didn't feel comfortable explaining it to the nurse.

Denial is a part of dissociation. Underneath denial may be what is referred to as *psychosomatic symptoms*. Psychosomatic symptoms refer to physiological and physical symptoms that are related to a mental or emotional response. When a person goes to a physician for pain, the doctor may not find any physical reason for the pain; in such a case, the pain might be determined to be psychosomatic. Levine and Frederick explain:

> Trauma can make a person blind, mute, or deaf; it can cause paralysis in legs, arms, or both; it can bring about chronic neck and back pain, chronic fatigue syndrome, bronchitis, asthma, gastrointestinal problems, severe PMS, migraines, and a whole host of so-called psychosomatic conditions. Any physical system capable of binding the undischarged arousal caused by trauma is fair game. The trapped energy will use any aspect of our physiology available to it.[13]

In other words, we may express our pain through our bodies, despite the lack of any physical causation for the pain.

Psychosomatic symptoms and/or PTSD are commonly caused by rape. Recently I have seen several female clients who experienced date rape. This event can affect the woman indefinitely and can cause problems in all areas of her life. Combat trauma is another major cause of PTSD. It too can show up as psychosomatic illness if there are no physical injuries.

Traumatic anxiety is another symptom of trauma.[14] This anxiety is much more profound than the general anxiety that is usually experienced by an individual. Traumatic anxiety can include an elevated arousal state, symptoms of trauma, and immobility. With this type of anxiety comes a nagging awareness that something is wrong—an anxiety that is almost constant. The traumatic anxiety displays itself as nervousness, fretting and worrying, and in appearing to be "high-strung." The sufferer frequently experiences panic, dread, and highly over-dramatized reactions to trivial events. These maladies are not permanent fixtures of the personality, but are indicative of a nervous system temporarily, though perpetually, overwhelmed.[15]

All of the trauma symptoms listed above have been treated effectively with EMDR. In her 2001 book, *Eye Movement Desensitization Reprocessing: Basic Principles, Protocols, and Procedure*, Shapiro asserts that the goal of EMDR is to "rapidly metabolize the dysfunctional residue from the past and transform it into something useful."[16] Although her whole book explains this statement, it is helpful to note that EMDR will take a client back to the original trauma, either through image or sensation. While the memory that created the imbalance in the nervous system is accessed, the EMDR process is used to transmute the negative experiences into adaptive learning experiences.

If you choose to experience this healing modality, find a therapist who is trained in EMDR. Although you generally do not need to relive the original trauma, memories may surface. It is helpful to have a support system during the time you use this process. The therapist will help you assess your need for support. He or she will use some exercises to help strengthen your inner resources. Examples of resources are friends, hobbies, family, inspirational books, and inner resources such as the ability to calm yourself, a meditation or yoga practice, or just the ability to change your thinking to something positive when you become overwhelmed with emotion or images.

It is essential to identify and clear not only the symptoms but also the underlying issue that caused the symptoms. During the EMDR process, the therapist will help you identify beliefs such as *negative cognitions* (NC) and *positive cognitions* (PC).

Beliefs you hold about yourself regarding the trauma repeat in other current situations as well. The belief is often one that is stored below your conscious awareness and permeates your daily life. Accessing this negative belief and bringing the awareness out into the open helps you to recognize how your behaviors have supported it. This recognition will bring you more choices in life. As stated above, the therapist will also help you to identify a positive cognition. This positive cognition, or new belief, allows you to replace the negative belief with something positive. Even the process of identifying the negative belief and thinking about what would be the appropriate replacement belief is supportive of healing.

When using EMDR, the therapist will either use eye movement, hand pulsers, or headphones with sound. The process brings the client's attention from one side of the brain to the other and back and forth. With eye movement, this can be done by watching the therapist's fingers as he or she moves them from one side to the other in front of your eyes. With a light bar, you follow the lights as they move from left to right and back, over and over for about thirty seconds at a time. With hand pulsers, the pulsers vibrate lightly from one hand to the next and then back and forth. With headphones, sound tones move from one ear to the other and back and forth. This process, no matter the tool used, is called bilateral stimulation (BLS).

The therapist will have the client start with a disturbing image and will then facilitate several thirty-second sessions of bilateral stimulation. During the break in processing, the client will take a deep breath and release the image (energy) and then continue again. I see this as developing the imagination muscle and allowing the body-mind to calm itself and relax. This process reduces the negative effect of the target or original image, lessening the impact of the memory and allowing the client to gain a sense of control.

There is a variation to this process, which is when the therapist uses her or his hands to tap lightly on the client's knee—first one and then the other, back and forth—creating the same stimulation. In between sessions with the therapist, the client can do this alone to experience calmness when images surface.

Shapiro offers a great example of how this works. Doug was a counselor at a Veterans Outreach program who had served in Vietnam. He had a traumatic memory that kept resurfacing. Shapiro was able to have Doug hold the traumatic memory of a buddy giving him upsetting news while he was unloading dead soldiers from a rescue helicopter during the war. At the same time, Shapiro used BLS, prompting Doug's memory to change. After several sets of the BLS, Doug no longer had the auditory part of the memory. After further sets, he imaged the experience as looking like a paint chip under water, and he reported feeling calm and as though he could tell everybody to go home—the war was over. Later, when he was asked to think of Vietnam, the image that came was that of the country looking like a garden paradise when he first flew over it. Shapiro checked with Doug months later, and the traumatic memory was still clear.[17]

Shapiro's success confirmed that decade-old memories could be accessed and resolved through EMDR. This discovery motivated Shapiro to continue exploring the technique; she conducted a controlled study with twenty-two victims of rape, molestation, or combat in Vietnam. All of these proved successful as well.[18]

Trauma and dissociation can create major blocks to developmental tasks, and the people who experience them are often disconnected from their bodies in some manner. One way to resolve health issues is to help people reconnect with their bodies. A part of the EMDR process known as the *body scan* can be helpful in bringing a client back into his or her body.[19] After the processing is complete, the therapist will have the client scan her or his body from the top of the head downward, noticing if there is any "tension, tightness or unusual sensation" related to the relevant issue.[20]

In my experience with this practice, clients have indeed noticed sensations. With more BLS, the sensations move, change, or go away. The process is continued until the sensations are cleared, even in the next session if necessary. Many clients have used this process on their own to pay attention to pain or sensations, and by tapping on their knees (right and then left) to the rhythm of a heartbeat, they can clear their own pain.

If I sound like an advocate for EMDR, there's a good reason: it works. In my graduate work at Gonzaga University, I studied Carl Jung and dream work, which proved meaningful and rewarding. Later I trained in a cognitive-behavioral approach with the William Glasser Institute. [21] Today, whenever I am treating trauma and deem it appropriate, I use hypnosis or EMDR. I often use hypnosis for strengthening new behaviors and EMDR for clearing trauma.

Several months ago, I had a regular client come into my office, shaken and stunned. I work by the Spokane River, and on her way to my office, the client witnessed police cars, an ambulance, and a fire truck responding to a man who had jumped off the Monroe Street Bridge into the river. I had her sit down, and I began bilateral stimulation (BLS) on her knees immediately. Within a few moments, the image was neutralized and we could go on with our regular session. Had this technique not been available, she might have been traumatized for months.

After Hurricane Katrina hit New Orleans in 2005, numerous hurricane victims were sent to Houston, TX, and one of my therapist friends was subsequently sent there by his agency to help. My first thought was that the victims would be stunned and in the denial part of grief. As such, I believed they would be unable to obtain much help from counselors in the early stages of their trauma. When my friend returned, he reported that the situation was indeed chaotic and that he hadn't been able to offer effective help. I believe calling EMDRIA would have been more helpful. The EMDR International Association (EMDRIA) is a membership organization of mental health professionals who, in part, volunteer to travel to areas in need, helping with traumatic situations.[22] Administering BLS would have helped clear the immediate trauma so that it would not continue to resurface in the victims' lives.

When you think about trauma, dissociation, and psychosomatic symptoms, remember that self-healing is cooperating with the natural healing process. Shapiro explains:

> Inherent in the Adaptive Information Processing Model [EMDR] is the concept of psychological self-healing, a construct based on the body's healing response to physical injury. For instance, when you cut your hand, your body works to close and heal the wound. If something blocks the healing, such as a foreign object or repeated trauma, the wound will fester and cause pain. If the block is removed, healing will resume. A similar sequence of events seems to occur with mental processes. That is, the natural tendency of the brain's information-processing system is to move toward a state of mental health. However, if the system is blocked or becomes imbalanced by the impact of a trauma, maladaptive responses are observed. These responses may be triggered by present stimuli or perhaps by the attempt of the information-processing mechanism to resolve the material.[23]

With this in mind, although the focus of this book is self-healing, and I am showing that our bodies move into self-healing, it is important to remember that self-healing does not mean doing everything yourself. Just as you would refer a loved one to someone who could be helpful, guide yourself to those who have the training and appropriate modalities to help you in your own self-healing process.

Tools and Exercises

1. Write notes in your journal in response to the questions listed previously regarding the DSM-IV-TR definition of posttraumatic stress disorder (PTSD).

2. Check out the Symptoms of Trauma in appendix 4, and list the symptoms you have.

3. Take the Trauma Questionnaire in appendix 5. If you find you have several of these experiences, it is important that you contact a counselor in your area who treats PTSD.

4. Write a list of traumas that you have experienced in your life. Identify the *big T's* and the *little t's*. On a scale of 1–10, with 10 being the most disturbing, rate how disturbing each trauma is for you now. If you have traumas that are 5 or higher, you may want to check **http:// www.emdr.com** to see if there are therapists certified in EMDR available in your area. Take this book with you and share with the therapist that you are in the process of healing your pain.

5. After taking the Trauma Questionnaire, if you believe you may have been sexually abused, call your local mental health center. They can provide you with local counselors to assist you. If you have health insurance, you can also check the counselors available to you under your plan. Most counselors list the areas in which they specialize.

6. List some beliefs you may have stored in your mind that you would like to change, such as, "I am unlovable," "I have to suffer," "Things always go wrong for me," and "I have to do it all myself." Relax and see if you can think back to the first time you remember thinking this. What was the situation? What positive belief would replace the negative belief? Write about it in your journal.

7. You may not have the trauma you are reading about but know someone who has. Take some time to talk with your friend and educate her or him about PTSD and the resources available as listed in this book.

8. Spend time awakening your body. You can do this through bodywork. You may want to receive massage, reflexology, or an energy medicine session such as Reiki or Touch for Health.[24] You might also take a slow, gentle, yoga class that nurtures and supports you. You can build up to a more advanced class, but begin slow.

9. Some believe that when you experience trauma, you lose a part of your soul. Many years ago, from a shaman who would like to remain unknown, I learned to do a process called *soul retrieval*. This process may help you to bring back the parts of yourself that have split off during a traumatic experience. Close your eyes and focus in your heart. Bring your attention above the top of your head, out of the crown chakra and up into the heavens. Ask God, your Creator, or your

Source to find any parts of yourself that have been split off, lost, or separated from you. Ask that these parts of you be cleansed in the Light of Love and returned to you. Ask for the cleansing of any elements you have taken on that do not belong to you, and ask that they be returned to the person to whom they belong. Allow yourself some time to experience this process, and when you are complete, thank God, your Creator, or your Source, and come back into the room. Feel the difference, and drink a glass of water.

Week Ten: Your Energy System

In the last few weeks, we explored your beliefs and feelings, as well as how to handle trauma. Now we will explore your energy system. At some level, you are already aware of subtle energies. Let's look more consciously at these energies and learn about some tools for working with them that will assist you on the road to self-healing.

As I just noted, all of us at times feel subtle energy. You may have walked into a room and immediately sensed that there was someone there before you who was angry. Maybe you have been around someone who was depressed and noticed that you began to lose energy and feel unmotivated as well. Have you ever been in a room full of people and seen someone across the room looking at you ... and you then felt a surge of energy and excitement? How about spending time with young children and being energized by the experience? Subtle energy is the energy around your body. It is a part of you, and it is felt by others as well.

In his 1998 book, *Subtle Energy*, William Collinge tells us that Albert Einstein showed through physics what the sages have taught for thousands of years.[1] Every animate and inanimate object in our material world is made of energy, and everything radiates energy. The earth is one enormous energy field; in fact, it is a field of fields. The human body, a microcosm of this, is a constellation of many interacting and interpenetrating energy fields.[2]

You may have heard others talk about subtle energy around the body. Collinge gives the example of an 81-year-old woman named Maggie in a retirement village whose physical exam showed she had recently made great progress in her health. When Collinge questioned her, he learned the only difference in her life was that she had been caring for her daughter's dog for a few months.[3]

Although it is common knowledge that having a pet is beneficial to the health of elderly people living alone (and all of us), researchers at the Institute of HeartMath in Boulder Creek, California, have found that feelings of love and tenderness affect the heart energetically.[4] The heart is by far the most powerful of several energy centers in the body. When feelings of caring and love are accessed, the beating pattern of the heart shifts to move in a more even and regular capacity. This in turn alters the electromagnetic field of the heart, which then brings tremendous benefits to the person on all levels—body, mind, and spirit.[5]

Collinge explained, "The dog didn't soothe Maggie's heart; she did it herself by accessing these feelings."[6] What a great example of self-healing!

It is helpful to understand how affected we are by the energetic field around us. Collinge gives examples of how energy is felt and how it changes. One example describes the energy between a mother and child. Although there is an emotional connection, there is also a familiar energetic connection as well.[7] A mother can be comforting to a child in ways others cannot. Additionally, those who pray together share an energetic connection, and "every spiritual tradition has a way of accounting for the energetic phenomena that occur during devoted spiritual practice."[8] Collinge notes that at a silent spiritual retreat, an individual may experience an explosion of light behind the eyes; another individual at a church service may be overcome by the Holy Spirit and respond by laughing or crying uncontrollably.[9]

Another example from Collinge is that of a mental health therapist who "starts each day with plenty of energy but feels dragged out and depleted at the end. She decided to learn more about energy and took a class in *Chi kung*, an ancient Chinese tradition of energy cultivation."[10] She found one of the principles to be the notion that "when you touch another person there is an exchange in energy" and that "energy will move from the person with the highest energy to the one with the lowest energy."[11] The therapist experimented with this and found that her teacher was correct. When she stopped touching her clients, she stopped losing her own vital energy.[12]

Collinge gives another interesting example: "A group of Benedictine monks who had been chanting daily for years suddenly stopped practice. Soon thereafter they began experiencing low energy, sleep disorders, and other health problems. All their symptoms disappeared when chanting practice was reinstated." Collinge observes, "Chanting affects our energetic anatomy on several levels, from the electrical potential of our brain to the energy passing through energy centers throughout our body." He adds that Gregorian chant music "can serve as a delightful means of self-generation of energy."[13]

I remember when I worked at the Healing Lodge of the Seven Nations as a mental health counselor. This was a treatment program for adolescent men and women, primarily Native Americans. After spending all day with their high and low energies, as well as their manic and depressive moods, I felt unusually tired after work. Often, I would go straight to my daughter's house and roll around with my young grandchildren. After a few minutes with them, my energy level lifted, and I was able to go on with the rest of my day.

In addition to the subtle energies in and around our bodies, we are affected by the subtle energies of the world around us. Collinge shares that there are studies showing an increase in mental hospital admissions, suicides, and even lottery payouts related to the cycles of the moon.[14] The planet radiates its own energy, and cosmic happenings can affect our behavior on a daily basis. Scientists know some of these energies, such as the geomagnetic field, but others are left to esoteric tradition.[15]

One response to these energy patterns is *feng shui* (pronounced fung-shway). Feng shui is an ancient Chinese art involving the placement of objects in such a way that energy can flow smoothly, thereby allowing health, peace, and prosperity to come to those who inhabit the space.

Feng means "wind," and *shui* means "water." In Chinese culture, gentle wind and clear water have always been associated with good harvest and good health. Thus, "good feng shui" came to mean good livelihood and fortune, while "bad feng shui" came to mean hardship and misfortune.

According to Rodika Tchi, a Feng Shui consultant, "Feng Shui is based on the Taoist vision and understanding of nature, particularly on the idea that the land is alive and filled with Chi, or energy." She explains that in ancient times, Chinese people believed that the energy of the land and the way that energy flowed were strong determinants of the kingdom's fate. The Taoist theory of yin and yang, or opposing but complementary opposites, and the five elements of Feng Shui—wood, fire, earth, metal and water— are primary underpinnings of this theory. Light and color are also believed to be very important.[16]

Tchi further explains that the main tools used in a feng shui analysis are the *compass* and the *bagua*. The bagua is an octagonal grid containing the symbols of the I Ching, the ancient oracle on which feng shui is based. Knowing the bagua of your home will help you understand the connection of specific feng shui areas of your home to specific areas of your life.[17]

I have created a bagua map for you to reference on my website and in appendix 6. Look at the map from the direction in which you enter the room. You can then place items that will attract energy to the areas where you would like more energy. Many books have been written about feng shui, and there are many different styles of this ancient science. Feng shui is about bringing harmony to an area. Some of the ways to do this include removing clutter, making adjustments for rooms and homes that are irregularly shaped, harmonizing with color, and using tools for abundance and purification.

This is a very basic introduction to feng shui. I strongly encourage you to research this fascinating topic on your own. That being said, I have had some validating experiences with it myself. Several years ago I was looking for a home to buy. I wanted to be near water and found a nice house north of Spokane with a beautiful creek nearby. As I walked the property, I realized that the house had been built between two small hills in a canyon, and there was no place for the energy to move. I saw that energy would get stuck between the two hills, right where the house was built.

I informed the realtor, "According to feng shui, the energy here would get stuck around the house. That would mean whoever lived here would get sick." He looked at me with surprise and described the illnesses of the two people who lived there. He explained that these illnesses were occasioning their move. While this was sad for me to hear, I was not proficient in feng shui and didn't understand how to remedy the situation.

Later, when I did purchase a home across from the Spokane River, I had a feng shui practitioner come over to help me make sure the space was able to attract good chi and allow the energy to flow easily. She was very helpful when I was building my office. She instructed me to make a flat wall where a corner would have been. This revision eliminated a sharp corner that would have been pointing at me when I sat in my chair. It also offered me more room. I've had several additional good experiences using feng shui, but the one I would like to share here took place while seeing a new massage therapist.

When I went into her office and rested my body on her table, I felt extremely uncomfortable. I was face down and felt the energy above me as disturbing. I sat up, looked up, and saw that she had a three-dimensional metal star above the massage table. There was a sharp point coming right down toward the back of her customers. When she came into the room, I pointed this out to her. While not aware of feng shui and energy medicine, she kindly took the star down. As I write this, I can't help but wish I had followed up with her to see if she experienced a better return rate after making the change.

Collinge explains how technology offers some understanding of subtle energy, but that it is also important to note the human perceptual system is able to pick up energies that current technology has not yet been able to measure. Science tells us that if we cannot measure it, it does not exist, to which Collinge responds, "By this logic, of course, brain waves didn't exist until the invention of EEG equipment."[18]

To help you understand the subtle energies, I have included six principles described by Collinge.[19]

1. *We are beings of energy.* When we think of our anatomy, we ordinarily think of our bones,

muscles, organs, and other physical tissues. However, we also have an energetic anatomy. It is composed of multiple interacting energy fields that envelop and penetrate our physical body, govern its functioning, and extend out into the world around us. This anatomy serves as a vehicle for the circulation of vital energies that enliven and animate our lives.

2. *The earth herself has an energetic anatomy, similar to our own, that influences our own energy field.* The entire earth and biosphere in which we live is one gigantic living organism, with its own metabolic and energetic qualities. Energy centers, energy channels, and energy fields emanating from the earth, plants, and animals are in many ways analogous to our own. By understanding this vast system's energetic life, of which we are a part, we can learn to live in a greater state of harmony and balance.

3. *Our relationships with other people are shaped by the interactions of our energies.* Our relationships are based on more than just psychology and family history. The energetic states that we bring to one another can introduce dynamics that are even more profoundly influential. Simply by touching another person, we influence what happens in that individual's energy field. We can come to understand the impact of our own energy on others, and theirs on us, so as to relate with great clarity and effectiveness.

4. *Through the simple act of breathing, we traverse the boundary between the physical and the spiritual at every moment.* There is no life activity more important than breathing. It is our most immediate and intimate connection to the life force in every moment of our lives. It is a direct link to many expressions of subtle energy and spiritual attunement, as well as a doorway to profound states of harmony and peace.

5. *We are each capable of sustaining and cultivating our vital energy.* Our vital energy has a metabolism that we can come to understand and manage. Through attending to the nourishment we take into our bodies, our patterns of rest and activity, and our practice of energy cultivation disciplines, we can learn to become the stewards of our vital energy.

6. *Meditation, prayer, and healing are rich with subtle energy phenomena that represent contact with the spiritual dimension.* Many experiences we have during these practices can be taken as direct evidence of a state of communion or communication with Spirit. Healing abilities are present within us all, and we have unknowingly used them throughout our lives.[20]

Biofield

Several different words are used for the energy around your body. In China it is called *chi*, in Japan it is called *ki*, and in metaphysical circles in the US, it has been known as the *aura*. Researchers like Richard Pavek, originally of the Biofield Institute, refer to this energy as the *biofield*.[21] At mind-body expos, I have seen people taking aura photographs. These photos show the electromagnetic field around your body, which is actually comprised of several layers of energy, a phenomenon referred to as the *etheric field*. There are many descriptions of the etheric field, which differ somewhat from one another. When thinking about this energetic field, imagine the closest layer around the body resembling the shape of the body, and the next layer being similar in shape but farther away, and on and on, much like an outline around the body, layer after layer.

Collinge explains that the first layer is called the vital layer or *thermal body*; photos taken with infrared cameras can make this layer visible.[22] The second is the *emotional body*, which is generally described as the zone of feelings around us. Third is the *mental* or *causal body*, where our mental workings and visual imaginings reside. Fourth is the *astral body*, which has long been correlated with intuition and the heart. Fifth is the *etheric template*, which contains the data necessary to create the etheric body in perfect form. Sixth is the *celestial body*, and seventh is the *ketheric body;* both of these are connected to spiritual consonance. Collinge explains the reason this is important is that we need to understand our body is "encased within, and fully penetrated by, an energy field that influences what happens on the physical level."[23] He adds that the biofield's influence on what happens in our physical body "is well proven by studies of energy healing, such as Therapeutic Touch, a form of healing in which the practitioner touches only the energy field of the recipient and not the physical body."[24] I will discuss this further later on, when I introduce you to Reiki.

As we look at the biofield, you may remember a story of mine in the beginning of this book. Part of my motivation to embrace the concept of prevention in self-healing came from wearing a necklace from Biopro, now Gia Wellness. This company makes products that protect the energetic biofield around your body from negative influences that come from cell phones, televisions, microwaves, and so forth. This experience for me is a testament to the fact that some people are more sensitive than others and are therefore more affected by our environment. I will share more about this in Week Twelve. It also taught me that prevention is an important part of self-healing. This information is helpful as we explore healing modalities that will help you with your self-healing.

Chakras

I introduced you to chakras earlier in the book when talking about life purpose and intuitive readings. Now I'd like to share more about these energy centers that store such valuable information.

Chakras are energy centers in the body within our subtle bodies. The word *chakra* means "wheel" in Sanskrit. The chakras appear to function as energy transformers, taking the higher level of energy in our subtle body and bringing it into a lower level of energy, which is then translated into hormonal, physiologic, and cellular changes throughout the body. The chakras connect with each other and with the physical cellular structure of the body by fine subtle energy channels called *nadis*.[25] The Hindu system recognizes numerous chakras or energy centers, but I usually work with the seven main ones located along the spine. I have been intuitively reading the information in chakras for over thirteen years now. More recently, an eighth chakra is appearing to me; in it, I read karmic information.

Aligned along the spine, the chakras run from the base of the spine to above the head. Each major chakra is associated with a major nerve plexus and a major endocrine gland. I will give you an overview of each and then go into more detail. To visualize them, see Figure 5.

Chakra One: Coccygeal associated with the sacral-coccygeal nerve plexus governing the reproductive system and the gonads in the endocrine system.[26] The information contained in the first chakra relates to survival, being in a physical body, safety, security, the ability to stand up for oneself, tribal information, and information relating to the material world.

Chakra Two: Sacral associated with the sacral nerve plexus governing the genitourinary system and the leydig in the endocrine system.[27] The information contained in the second chakra relates to relationships, emotions, intimacy, sexuality, creativity, work, and money.

Chakra Three: Solar plexus associated with the solar nerve plexus governing the digestive system and the adrenals in the endocrine system.[28] The information contained in the third chakra relates to vitality, energy distribution, inner strength, self-control, power, ego, personality, desire, care of self and others, and self-esteem.

Chakra Four: Heart associated with the heart nerve plexus governing the circulatory system and the thymus in the endocrine system.[29] The information contained in the fourth chakra relates to love, self-love, love of others, love of God, affinity, loneliness and commitment, forgiveness and compassion, as well as hope and trust.

Chakra Five: Throat associated with the cervical ganglia medulla nerve plexus governing the respiratory system and the thyroid in the endocrine system.[30] The information contained in the fifth chakra relates to communication, choice, strength of will, capacity to make decisions, speech, individual needs, and self-expression.

Chakra Six: Third eye associated with the hypothalamus pituitary nerve plexus governing the autonomic nervous system and the pituitary in the endocrine system.[31] The information contained in the sixth chakra relates to insight, clear seeing, clairvoyance, intuition, self-evaluation, intellect, intuition, and wisdom.

Chakra Seven: Head associated with the cerebral cortex pineal nerve plexus governing the CNS central control system and the pineal in the endocrine system.[32] The information contained in the seventh chakra relates to consciousness, knowingness, values, ethics, courage, selflessness, faith and inspiration, spirituality, and devotion.

Below, I have listed more details about the chakras. This is an overview and gives some examples of how you may bring your body/mind/spirit into balance. This information may help you to determine where you are out of balance. This is just an overview, and you may want to check the bibliography, particularly Anodea Judith's 1997 book, *Eastern Body, Western Mind,* for more information.[33]

Chakra One

Orientation: Self-preservation.[34]

Chakra one is about your foundation and survival. The information contained within this chakra relates to being in your body and becoming independent and self-sufficient. This chakra is connected to your immune system.

Issues of the first chakra include "roots, grounding, nourishment, trust, health, home, family, prosperity and abundance."[35]

Signs of Deficiency in the First Chakra:

- Feeling disconnected from your body
- Difficulty maintaining a healthy weight (underweight)
- Feelings of fear, anxiety, and difficulty settling
- Difficulty focusing and following through
- Difficulty with finances
- Poor boundaries (see Week Five on boundaries)[36]

Signs of Excess in the First Chakra:

- Overeating and obesity
- Hoarding and greed
- Overly focused on material possessions
- Feeling lazy, tired, fatigued
- Fear of change
- High need for security
- Rigid boundaries[37]

The imbalance of the subtle energy around the body shows up in the chakras. Remember, they are like computers that receive and analyze all information that comes in. This imbalance affects us emotionally and ultimately affects the physical health of the body. Caroline Myss outlines emotional issues that are related to the first chakra. They are listed below.[38]

- Inability to feel safe, secure, and trusting
- Inability to provide for oneself and others, to prosper
- Inability to stand up for oneself, to be grounded in clear beliefs
- Inability to feel settled, nest, and feel safe and connected to home
- Lack of connection with social norms, laws, and order
- Depression and/or anxiety

Health Issues That May Arise from First Chakra Imbalances:

- Immune related disorders
- Frequent illness
- Eating disorders such as obesity or anorexia
- Disorders of the bones and teeth
- Disorders of the bowel, anus, and large intestine, such as rectal tumors and cancer
- Problems with the legs, including varicose veins
- Lower back pain and sciatica
- Problems with the base of the spine, buttocks, legs, knees, and feet

I met a young man at a workshop I facilitated in Ireland in 2008. He appeared to be anxious and nervous. In sitting down to read him intuitively, I became immediately aware that I could not detect a grounding cord at all. I looked at his first chakra and saw an image of it being blown out, as if there were no chakra there whatsoever. I asked him, "What happened to you on the day you were born?" He looked at me with wide eyes and shock.

He said, "My mother died." I could see that this event had created great distress in terms of his being in a physical body, and he had suffered all his life. Using my hands, I was able to move the energy around his body and through his chakras to re-establish his connection with Mother Earth and to repair his chakra. Afterward, he appeared much calmer. When I left him, I thought that perhaps this was the main reason I had gone to Ireland—to help this young man feel stable again.

To help balance the first chakra, sit and image a grounding cord going down from the base of your spine into the center of the earth, as recommended by Mary Ellen Flora in *Chakras: Key to Spiritual Opening*.[39] This grounding cord can be like a waterfall, a tree trunk, or a beam of light. Sense the grounding cord going down all the way through our planet to the fiery center of Mother Earth. Release energy down your grounding cord. Start at the top of your head, releasing energy down your neck and the channels on either side of your spine, all the way down your grounding cord to the center of the earth. Take a deep breath and continue to release energy, keeping this grounding cord attached near the base of your spine and the center of the earth. With practice, you will begin to stay grounded.

The following are additional grounding exercises to help balance the first chakra:

1. Spend some time in nature. Be around the trees or the water. Sit yourself down on the earth and breathe. Take off your shoes and feel the earth under your feet.

2. For calming and self-soothing, bilateral stimulation (BLS) is helpful as discussed earlier in the section on EMDR. With your fingertips, tap gently on the outside of your right leg and then on the outside of your left leg; continue to do so, moving back and forth. Alternatively, you can do this on the top of your thighs. The tapping can be done at the pace of your heartbeat (da dum ... da dum ...). These taps on your legs are called puppy pats. You can also cross your arms gently around your chest and tap on one arm and then the other.

3. Eating root vegetables is helpful for grounding. Organic vegetables are best because they take their nutrients from the soil in which they are grown. Grilled and roasted root vegetables are healthy and delicious. Protein-rich meals in general are grounding.

4. Exercise is helpful for grounding. Be aware of being in your body when you exercise, be aware of the bottom of your feet when you walk or run, and hold your awareness in each movement when you do aerobics or dance. Yoga, tai chi, and Qigong are all helpful for grounding.

5. Receiving in a healthy way is very important to first chakra healing. Allow yourself to partake in massage, Reiki, or reflexology. If you have difficulty allowing yourself to be touched, find a massage therapist who specializes in working with clients who have abandonment or abuse issues from childhood. You can also receive Therapeutic Touch or Reiki and ask that the therapist work in your energy field—but without touching you. Cuddle with a good friend, spouse, lover, child, grandchild, or treasured pet.

Chakra Two

Orientation: Self-gratification

The second chakra is the sacral chakra, associated with sensual movement, connection, and sexuality. The information contained in the second chakra relates to relationships, emotions, intimacy, sexuality, creativity, work, and money.

Issues of the second chakra include movement, sensation, emotions, sexuality, desire, need, and pleasure.[40]

Signs of Deficiency in the Second Chakra:

• Holding the body rigid and having rigid attitudes and beliefs
• Frigidity
• Poor social skills
• Denial of pleasure
• Rigid or excessive boundaries

- Fear of change
- Lack of desire, passion, and excitement

Signs of Excess in the Second Chakra:

- Sexual addiction
- Addition to food, alcohol, drugs, shopping, etc.
- Avoidance of responsibility
- Overwhelmed and ruled by emotions (hysteria, mood swings, drama junkies)
- Emotionally sensitive
- No or few boundaries, invasive of others
- Seductive manipulation
- Codependent
- Obsessive attachment

Myss also outlines emotional and mental issues related to the second chakra. They are listed below:[41]

- Issues of power and control
- Excessive blaming
- Excessive guilt
- Lack of creativity or excessive creativity and not functioning in daily needs
- Money issues
- Issues related to sexual activity (promiscuity, frigidity, etc.)
- Issues related to ethical behavior

Health Issues That May Arise from Second Chakra Imbalances:

- Health issues related to the reproductive organs
- Disorders of the spleen and urinary system
- Menstrual difficulties, PMS (Premenstrual Syndrome), and PMDD (Premenstrual Dsyphoric Disorder)
- Sexual dysfunction
- Chronic lower back pain, sciatica
- Inflexibility of joints
- Loss of sensual pleasure (food, sex, other interests)

Women and men who have been sexually abused may have some blockage in this chakra. Once, while teaching a Reiki I class, I saw this with a client. In using Reiki, a form of hands-on healing, we use the chakra centers as a guide for where to lay our hands. When placing hands on or above the second chakra, a few inches below the belly button, the healing was directed toward the areas listed in the health section above. When I placed my hands on my client's second chakra area as a demonstration, I could feel an incredible amount of energy in them to the point that my hands started to ache. I looked at my client and she began to tear up, looking at me as if she were frightened. I saw in my mind an image of her being sexually abused as a child. I encouraged her to let herself feel her feelings and to cry, assuring her that I would assist her by moving the energy in the chakra. She said, "I can't."

Understand that in addition to some of the other healings I facilitate, I have at times been a vessel for moving energy from my clients through me as a release. This is a shamanic technique that I have not learned; instead, it came to me in my journey as an energy healer. That said, I asked the client mentioned above if I could move the pain. She agreed to it, and I immediately became a conduit for the energy and cleared the block for her. I started shaking and crying, not moving around, but as if I were in deep pain. I cleared this pain through myself, and afterward I didn't feel anything. I didn't feel as if I had been in pain or had cried. My client looked relaxed, and the pain appeared to have cleared. She agreed that it had, and we used this as an example of another healing modality in the class.

It's important to note that I don't use this technique often, and I do not teach it to my clients. For me it usually happens spontaneously, and I don't fight it. My students are all metaphysically oriented and open to this information, so they were not afraid. The woman was grateful and able to begin practicing on other students. There were a few who had been sexually abused as children, and this was a good time for us to discuss how to respond to this issue with our Reiki clients.

I've listed some second chakra tools below that bring pleasure, nurturance, and healing balance to the body.

1. As with the first chakra, grounding is important in the second chakra. Movement is inherent in the workings of this chakra and can aid grounding. Gently moving to music is a self-nurturing way to get connected to your body and to ground. I particularly like Gabrielle Roth's music for this

purpose.[42] Gentle yoga, Qigong, and tai chi are also helpful for grounding.

2. Feel your feelings. So often in our culture we are taught to apologize when we find ourselves crying or expressing feelings. It is important to feel your feelings when they come up. It is not necessary to apologize for them or to understand why you are feeling what you are feeling. When you feel like crying, cry. When you are angry, feel the anger, notice that you are experiencing anger, and feel the feelings. When we feel our feelings, they go away.

3. Journaling with your inner self or your inner child is extremely helpful to heal the issues of the second chakra. Instead of finding yourself a fancy journal, get a simple, three-ring, spiral notebook in which you can scribble if you need or want. Write a letter to your inner self—the part of you that tries to get your attention but is often ignored because you are too busy or distracted to listen. Make a commitment to check in with yourself through a journal process daily. Set a timer for twenty minutes and journal whatever comes up. Even when you're not intentionally journaling, take notes from books you are reading, or jot down memories that surface in your daily life that you may want to examine later.

4. Boundary issues, which include weak boundaries and rigid boundaries, are affected by the second chakra. Become aware of your boundaries. Do you tend to stand too close to people, or are you

uncomfortable when touched? Do you share too much, or do you tend to keep your feelings to yourself? Do you have several friends but refrain from sharing your true feelings? Is your only close friend your cat or dog? Do you find you know more about your neighbors than the more intimate parts of yourself? You may want to check out my video on boundaries at **http://www.you tube.com/energymedicinedna**.

5. It's also important to allow yourself healthy pleasures. Journal to learn what you find pleasurable. Walk along the river, venture to the ocean, and take a long walk or an overnight trip to a nearby city. Rent three movies starring your favorite actress or actor and take a Sunday to have a cinematic binge. Get a massage, have a cup of aromatic tea in fine china, or visit your local museum. Explore something new, and begin to experience pleasure.

Chakra Three

Orientation: Self-definition.[43]

The third chakra is about transformation. This chakra governs the solar plexus, the digestive system, and the adrenals in the endocrine system. The information contained in the third chakra relates to vitality, energy distribution, inner strength, self-control, power, ego, personality, desire, care of self and others, and self-esteem.

Signs of Deficiency in the Third Chakra:

- Low energy
- Easily manipulated
- Poor self-discipline
- Low self-esteem
- Poor digestion
- Victim role
- Passive and blaming
- Unreliable

Signs of Excess in the Third Chakra:[44]

- Controlling
- Aggressive, dominating
- Needs to be right
- Stubborn
- Over-functioning and competitive
- Egotistical
- Hyperactive

Myss provides indications of emotional issues related to the third chakra:[45]

- Lack of trust
- Fearful and/or intimidating
- Low self-esteem, lack of self respect
- Inability to care for oneself in a healthy manner
- Sensitive to criticism
- Emotionally manipulating

- Enmeshment

Health Issues That May Arise from Third Chakra Imbalances:

- Eating disorders such as anorexia and bulimia
- Digestive disorders, indigestion, and ulcers
- Pancreatitis, hypoglycemia, and diabetes
- Gallbladder, liver disorders, and hepatitis
- Colon and intestinal problems
- Adrenal fatigue
- Muscle spasms and muscular disorders
- Chronic fatigue
- Hypertension

A physician friend who is a rheumatologist and immunologist was talking to me the other day about a client he had seen that morning. He shared his happiness to see the swelling in her hands' joints had gone down, and that other markers for her pain and illness had decreased substantially as well. However, he said that even with the progress, she kept stating she was getting worse. He was concerned about her but could not see anything to substantiate the concern, and he subsequently spent an unusually long time with her. At the end of the session, she brought out some papers she wanted him to sign that would give her an opportunity to file for disability. He related to me that he immediately felt very tired, and the rest of his day didn't go as well as usual.

When he was sharing this with me, I thought it might be a good time to introduce him to the concept of how energy gets drained in the third chakra. We talked about how his hope for her was high, and he had done well in prescribing the right treatment for her, but she didn't want it. Rather, she wanted him to determine she was disabled, when she was not. There was no way he could please her. This left him feeling disempowered. It was as though she had stolen his power. He and I had both been listening to and discussing Caroline Myss's series of CDs called *Energy Anatomy*, which is about the chakras, and we decided that his experience with this client was a fitting personal example of the sort of thing she describes.[46]

Below are some tools for the third chakra that bring self-esteem, power, and honor to the body:

1. Grounding is essential for all of the chakras. Explore Flora's and my grounding practices, as described in the tools for healing the first chakra.

2. Take a self-inventory. A simple practice of this at the end of the day before bed is to ask yourself what you did well and what you could have done better. I use this with my granddaughter when she stays with me. It is an excellent tool for children as well as adults.

3. Caroline Myss, author of *Anatomy of the Spirit*, suggests that you write down what you are doing that you know you should not be doing, and what you are not doing that you know you should be doing.[47] I have done this several times,

and it has always been extremely helpful and revealing.

4. Write out goals for your life. What do you want to accomplish in one year, five years, and ten years? A creative way to do this is to create a collage of pictures that represent what you want in your life. You can glue these pictures to a piece of cardboard and put the entire thing in a place you see often. Write out simple steps to achieve your goals. At the beginning of each month, check to see if you are on track. Bring consciousness to your desires and goals at the beginning of the month. The first day of each month has new energy, as does the first day of each week and the first day of each year.

5. The third chakra is about power and ego. Take a class in something you enjoy to increase your knowledge or ability. Read a book that will expand your awareness, knowledge, or skill. Join a group of others who have the same interest and support the direction in which you are moving.

6. Complete your unfinished projects. This is a fantastic way to unblock energy and increase your self-esteem. Take on one project a month, or one project a week for a month. Learn to finish what you begin. When I was a child, I was a Blue Bird, and we had Blue Bird promises we said every meeting. The only part of the pledge I remember is, "I promise to finish what I begin." Thinking of this often when I complete projects, I

fondly believe I remembered it because it was what I needed the most.

Chakra Four

Orientation: Self-acceptance[48]

The fourth chakra is associated with love and balance. It governs the circulatory system and the thymus in the endocrine system. The information contained in the fourth chakra relates to love, self-love, love of others, love of God, affinity, loneliness, commitment, hope, trust, as well as forgiveness and compassion.

Signs of Deficiency in the Fourth Chakra:[49]

- Being cold and withdrawn
- Being critical and judgmental
- Feeling isolated and lonely
- Depression
- Fear of intimacy, relationship problems
- Lacking empathy
- Narcissism

Signs of Excess in the Fourth Chakra:[50]

- Codependency (focusing on others rather than self)
- Having poor boundaries
- Being demanding of others
- Clinging to others

- Being jealous of others
- Behaving as a martyr

Myss outlines emotional issues related to the fourth chakra.[51] They are listed below:

- Mood swings
- Vacillating between loving and hating
- Grief and anger
- Self-centered behavior
- Loneliness
- Problems with commitment
- Inability to trust and forgive

Myss also notes health issues that may arise from fourth chakra imbalances, as follows:[52]

- Heart disease
- Lung cancer
- Bronchial pneumonia
- Sunken chest
- Shortness of breath
- Asthma and allergies
- Breast cancer
- Issues of the shoulders, upper back, and chest
- Immune system deficiency
- Problems with circulation

Several years ago when dating, I met a man who shared with me that he'd had four heart surgeries. Four heart surgeries! This man was in his forties! Well, being the mental health and energy therapist that I am, I talked with him about the fourth chakra. I asked what was happening with him in relationships that would have resulted in his heart having been "broken" four times. He denied any issues in this area but gave me a book that the last woman he dated had given him, *The Heart's Code*, written by Paul Pearsall.[53] The inside book jacket describes the book as "a fascinating synthesis of ancient wisdom, modern medicine, scientific research, and personal experience that proves that the human heart, not the brain, holds the secrets that link body, mind, and spirit." I looked at the book and was delighted to have found it. We decided not to continue dating, but the book was quite a gift.

Here are some tools and exercises that bring love and balance to the body. These tools can also be found in Flora's book, *Chakras: Key to Spiritual Opening*, as well as on my CD, *Chakra Clearing*.

1. Explore Flora's and my grounding practices, as described in the tools for healing the first chakra.

2. Breathing is an important part of loving your body and loving others. You may remember a time when you were holding a child and simply breathing together. Focusing on your own breath or focusing on breathing with another person are two wonderful ways to feel the life energy and the love in your heart. Deep breathing allows us to connect more deeply with our angels.

3. The practice of gratitude brings balance to the heart chakra. A great weekly practice is to write out twenty things for which you are grateful. It helps to do this the same time each week. For instance, you could do it every Monday morning. This gets the week off to a good start! You may find the same items coming up, but as you practice this exercise, you will find that your gratitude grows. I especially like this practice when I find myself feeling grumpy for no known reason. After writing my gratitude list, I always feel better. This is especially fun to do with children and grandchildren. It is a practice they will remember as they grow.

4. The heart chakra is about relationships. Relationships are always in a process of merging and separating. You may want to physically shift your body in movements of giving out and taking in. The Sun Salutation is a great exercise for this. You can perform an Internet search for it to learn more. Several websites show this yoga movement.

5. Journaling is especially helpful for this chakra. You can develop a relationship with yourself through the journal process. Here are some ways to use your journal; many of them are methods we've already discussed:

- Write a Dear God/Goddess letter, which is a letter expressing your thoughts and feelings to God/Goddess from your heart.
- Write a gratitude list.
- Write an anger letter. Use this as a way to vent and then let go. "I am so angry at … "
- When you find you are stuck, make a "To Do" list, and then reward yourself by using stickers or colored pens to check off what you accomplish.
- Write a list of pros and cons when you have difficulty making a decision.
- Write out your dreams. The book I love is *Realities of the Dreaming Mind*, by Swami Sivananda Rahda.[54]
- Write a prayer list. This can include prayers for yourself and for others.
- When you are reading a novel or self-help book, make notes in your journal when something moves you or awakens your senses, or when there is a "charge" connected to what you read. A "charge" is felt when you have a reaction—positive or negative. It may show up as resistance. Keeping notes while you read books gives you the ability to return to your journal and remember what was important to you.
- Write poetry or prose.

- Take a personal inventory. Write out what you did well today and what you didn't do well.

- Write out your priorities, which are the endeavors that are important for you to accomplish.

- Write what you love about your friends.

- Write what you love about yourself.

6. If you are in a marriage or an intimate relationship, you may want to get one journal and have each person write to the other in this journal. For example, the husband might write a morning message to his wife. Then, in the afternoon or evening, she would write a journal entry to him. Occasionally, the two can sit down and read the journal together. This practice is especially bonding in the beginning of a relationship, when communication tends to flow more easily. The goal of starting this at the beginning is to allow this pattern of communication to continue when issues arise. It is important to keep the lines of communication open. The practice can also renew a well-established relationship.

7. Many of us can benefit from the help of a counselor. Whether you have difficulty making and keeping friends, have unresolved grief, or have memories of childhood experiences that arise and create problems in your daily life, finding a counselor can help. There are many

modalities of therapy, and it is important to find the one that is best for you. For those who have experienced trauma (which is most of us), I recommend eye movement desensitization and reprogramming (EMDR). My experience with clients when using EMDR is that the technique allows them to clear trauma much more quickly than "talk therapy."

8. Although "discovery is not recovery," finding and reading appropriate books can help heal this chakra. Many books have exercises that help you learn and anchor the new behaviors. Check the endnotes section at the end of this book for ideas on other books to help in your journey.

Chakra Five

Orientation: Self-expression[55]

The fifth chakra is about communication and creativity. It is associated with the throat and the cervical ganglia medulla nerve plexus, which governs the respiratory system, as well as the thyroid in the endocrine system. The information contained in the fifth chakra relates to communication, choice, strength of will, capacity to make decisions, speech, individual needs, and self-expression.

Signs of Deficiency in the Fifth Chakra:

- Being introverted and shy
- Having a soft, weak voice
- Fear of speaking

- Difficulty using words appropriately
- Being especially secretive

Signs of Excess in the Fifth Chakra:

- Excessive talking
- Talking loudly and quickly, using talking as a defense
- Poor listening skills
- Gossiping
- Stuttering
- Interrupting others, inability to be silent

Again, Myss provides us with emotional and health issues, this time as they relate to the fifth chakra:[56]

- Inability to express oneself
- Indecisiveness
- Being critical and judgmental
- Having a lack of will
- Being dishonest and/or giving mixed messages

Health Issues That May Arise from Fifth Chakra Imbalances:

- Chronic sore throat
- Mouth ulcers
- Gum difficulties
- Throat cancer
- Laryngitis

- Joint problems
- Swollen glands
- Thyroid problems

Here are some tools that bring self-expression and creativity to the body:

1. Explore Flora's and my grounding practices, as described in the tools for healing the first chakra.

2. A great way to keep the throat chakra clear is through singing. Find some music you love and sing along. Sing loudly as well as softly, and play with the sound. Let it be fun.

3. Toning is also a great way to clear the fifth chakra. I remember about twenty years ago, while taking a bath, I realized I was getting sick. All of a sudden I felt feverish and ill. I intuitively began to tone, making sound deep from my belly. I did this for about ten minutes, just varying the sound, naturally following what felt right, and I was able to heal myself immediately. I later found a cassette tape by Steven Halpern that guided me through toning with the vowels.[57] I started practicing moving energy through my throat chakra using the sounds A ... E ... I ... O ... U. Use this same method to clear your fifth chakra starting with the A sound, toning quietly, and then getting louder, moving the tone up and down while feeling it in your whole body. I found that this not only clears the fifth chakra, but it also

clears the rest of the chakras. You can just focus on each chakra and then use sound to clear yourself.

4. Chanting is another way to clear the fifth chakra. There are many great chants available from many sources; find the chants that feel healing to your body.

5. Telling stories is another way to clear the fifth chakra. Talking with others from your heart is particularly helpful. Conversely, you may want to stop telling stories about negative things that have happened to you, if you find yourself telling the same negative story over and over again. Once you stop focusing on this story from the past, you will free up room for new energy in the present.

6. Journaling and automatic writing is also helpful in clearing the fifth chakra. When you journal, you may find that certain thoughts have a charge (an emotional response) or are significant. If so, read them aloud or share them with a friend. If something continues to come up over and over, you may want to read it repeatedly until it no longer has a charge for you.

Chakra Six

Orientation: Self-reflection[58]

The sixth chakra is about pattern recognition. It is associated with the third eye and the hypothalamus pituitary nerve plexus, which governs the autonomic nervous system, as well as the pituitary in the endocrine system. The information contained in the sixth chakra relates to insight, clear seeing, clairvoyance, intuition, self-evaluation, intellect, intuition, and wisdom.

Signs of Deficiency in the Sixth Chakra:

- Being insensitive to situations and others
- Poor vision, inability to see the future or image alternatives
- Difficulty visualizing
- Lack of imagination
- Poor memory
- Denial (unable to see what is happening)
- Rigid thinking, as in one way is the only way
- Inability to remember dreams

Signs of Excess in the Sixth Chakra:

- Hallucinations
- Obsessions
- Delusions
- Difficulty concentrating
- Nightmares

Myss provides the following emotional and health issues that correlate with the sixth chakra:[59]

- Inability (or resistance) to self-evaluate
- Difficulty with intellectual ability
- Feelings of inadequacy
- Close-mindedness
- Inability or unwillingness to learn from mistakes
- Incongruence between mental and emotional self-narratives

Health Issues That May Arise from Sixth Chakra Imbalances:

/

- Headaches
- Brain tumors, hemorrhage
- Stroke
- Neurological disturbances
- Blindness and deafness
- Full spinal difficulties
- Learning disabilities
- Seizures

Here are some tools that bring self-reflection and balance to the body. Remember to first explore Flora's and my grounding practices, as described in healing the other chakras.

1. Begin a dream journal, and be open to your dreams as a medium through which your Higher Self connects with you. There are several books on dream process. The one that I use is *Realities of the Dreaming Mind*, by Swami Sivananda Radha.[60] You may also find a local dream group, the

feedback of which could prove to be quite helpful, since healing in this chakra has much to do with opening the mind and being open to how others view us and our patterns.

2. Begin to notice when you become defensive, and write out the situation in your journal. You may begin to see a pattern. When you are defensive, ask yourself, "What am I defending? What am I afraid to see? What change may I have to make if I see this or believe this about myself?" Ask a trusted friend to help you view blocks that may be in the way of your seeing clearly. When I attended Doreen Virtue's Angel Practitioner Workshop in 2008, we practiced reading with partners.[61] At one point, Doreen asked us, "What is the question you are most afraid to ask Archangel Michael?" I was shocked by the answer that came to me, and it was the most powerful experience of the workshop!

3. Learn detachment. This is often a difficult challenge, but an extremely rewarding one. Practice observing situations as if they were on a movie screen. Don't push the image away or pull it toward you. Resist the urge to give advice or to fix or rescue. Watch situations play themselves out as you breathe and stay relaxed. Notice how easy your life becomes when detachment replaces reaction.

4. Hypnotherapy and visualization are extremely helpful for this chakra. My CD, *Chakra Clearing*, teaches you how to visualize as you clear your

chakras. You may also want to find a local hypnotherapist to guide you deeper into your imagination. There are many CDs that lead you in guided imagery as well. Explore your inner world through visualization in one of these ways.

5. Poor memory is a sixth chakra issue. You may want to find a simple book on memory that will help you to use word substitution, linking, or other association methods for improving memory. People sometimes forget things because they are not operating in present time. If you practice being in your body and in present time, you may find that your memory improves substantially. Be present, breathe, and be aware of what is happening within your body and around you at all times.

Chakra Seven

Orientation: Self-knowledge[62]

The seventh chakra is about understanding. It is located above the head and is associated with the cerebral cortex pineal nerve plexus, which governs the CNS central control system, as well as the pineal in the endocrine system. The information contained in the seventh chakra relates to consciousness, knowingness, values, ethics, courage, selflessness, faith and inspiration, spirituality, and devotion.

Signs of Deficiency in the Seventh Chakra:

- Learning difficulties

- Rigid belief systems
- Apathy
- Spiritual cynicism
- Overly focused on materialism, greed, and power over others
- Excess focus on being in a physical body, safety, security, money, work, relationships, and power

Signs of Excess in the Seventh Chakra

- Intellectualizing
- Spiritual addictions
- Confusion
- Dissociation from self and body
- Inability to stay present

Myss explicates issues of the heart and the body as they relate to the seventh chakra in the following two lists:

Emotional Issues Related to the Seventh Chakra:

- Inability to trust the life process
- Disruption in values and ethics
- Detachment from humanitarian issues
- Inability to see the larger picture
- Lack of faith
- Loss of purpose and meaning in life

Health Issues That May Arise from Seventh Chakra Imbalances:

- Extreme sensitivity to light, sound, and other environmental factors
- Spiritual depression (loss of meaning in life)
- Chronic exhaustion unrelated to physical disorders
- Migraines and headaches

As with each of the other chakras, first explore Flora's and my grounding practices (to reiterate, they are described in the tools for healing the first chakra). The following are some other tools that bring consciousness to the body:

1. There is an energy flow between all of the chakras, and they work together—each chakra affects the next. To help rebalance the body when the seventh chakra is in excess, focus on your body and your emotions. Practice scanning your body. Imagine a light, such as a flashlight, coming down from the top of your head inside your body. As this light flows in, notice different sensations in your body. Notice your feelings. You do not have to figure out why you feel what you are feeling … just notice it. You may notice tension in your shoulders. You may find that suddenly, when the light illuminates the heart, you feel sadness. Just feel the sensations and the feelings. Afterward, journal for ten to twenty minutes. Don't intellectualize and think about

what you are writing; just let the words flow from the pen.

2. If your seventh chakra is deficient, sit in a comfortable chair with a cup of tea or other nurturing beverage, and allow yourself to daydream. Go back to when you were a young child and remember your dreams. Many of us do not remember a lot of our childhood. If this is the case for you, do not allow it to discourage you. Think back to your dreams as a child or your activities. As you image this, think about what was important to you, and think about the things in which you believed. These can be discerned by reviewing your behavioral choices. Is there a part of yourself that you left behind and want to bring into your life today? Is there some aspect of the former ten-year-old that will inspire you? As an example, I remember that when I was young, about ten or eleven years old, I had an idea to write a cookbook. I had seen many recipes on the back of cereal boxes and other packages, so I wrote to companies like Quaker and Betty Crocker. They sent me recipes and glossy pictures. I had a purple, flowered suitcase full of these recipes and pictures. At that time, there was not an adult around who could have helped me with the next step, but many years later, as an adult, I saw a cookbook like the one I had envisioned—it was one that someone else had published. Although I don't cook much now, I do enjoy taking ideas and helpful tips and sharing them with others. My creativity now manifests as

sharing on my website, as well as in the classes and workshops I develop.

3. When you are feeling spiritually lost, it is often helpful to become activated by someone else's trust in God or the power of universal laws. You become activated by information that has a positive charge. You can find books or CDs by others who are spiritually connected. You even become activated by information as you read. An example from my own life came several years ago when a dear friend told me about *The Secrets of the Talking Jaguar*, by Martin Prechtel.[63] After I picked up the book at the library and began reading, I realized I had already read it. When I originally read it, I felt alive and energized, as if I was connecting with important ancient and spiritual guides. The second time I started reading it, the words were just black spots on the white page. I had already been activated to the vibration of this book, and it no longer raised my energy and vibration. You may want to go to a bookstore and find a book that evokes awareness within you that something big will happen—that you will be activated to the information in the Spirit of the book!

Tools and Exercises

This week has been full of tools and exercises. Take some time to assess where your chakras may be out of balance and intuitively decide which exercises would be best for you to practice. Over time, you may want to learn them all. However, I find it is better to learn one tool well and integrate it into your life. Once this has taken place, add another tool.

1. Review your week and see where you may have become more energized by the energy of others and where you may have been drained. Then, think back to your life before you suffered with pain. Who were the people in your life at that time? Were you energized or drained by them? What situations were you in that may have energized or drained you?

2. Use your journal to complete chakra sentence stems. This is where I begin the sentence for you, and you finish it with automatic writing. We've done a few of these already in this book, and I have created some more designed specifically for the chakras. Just let the words come directly onto the paper without thought. You may be amazed by what comes up! You will find some related specifically to the chakras in appendix 7: Chakra Stems.

Week Eleven: Energy Medicine

Kinesiology and Muscle Testing

One of the sources that really got me excited about kinesiology was the 2002 book, *Power vs. Force: The Hidden Determinants of Human Behavior*, by David R. Hawkins.[1] I heard about Dr. Hawkins previously when listening to a CD by Wayne Dyer entitled *A Spiritual Solution to Every Problem*, which I loved. In Week Ten, I shared about becoming activated by other people, and I was certainly activated by Dyer's CD.[2]

I can't help but digress here for a moment and share that I literally brushed up against Wayne Dyer today while waiting to get into the writer's workshop on a Hay House cruise to Alaska. Wayne had just finished his presentation to the group ahead of us, and I was delighted to see his smiling face and feel his positive energy as we came in contact.

Back on topic, at **http://dictionary.reference.com**, kinesiology is defined as "the science dealing with the interrelationship of the physiological processes and anatomy of the human body with respect to movement." In the forward to Dr. Hawkins's book, editor E. Whalen gives the history of kinesiology. I could not say it better, so I will quote him:

> The study of kinesiology first received scientific attention in the second half of the last century through the work of Dr. George Goodheart, who pioneered the specialty he called applied kinesiology after finding that benign physical stimuli — for instance, beneficial nutritional supplements — would increase the strength of certain indicator muscles, whereas hostile stimuli would cause those muscles to suddenly weaken. The implication was that at a level far below conceptual

consciousness, the body "knew," and through muscle testing was able to signal, what was good or bad for it. [Emphasis in original][3]

Whalen further explains, "Dr. John Diamond refined this specialty into a new discipline he called behavioral kinesiology."[4] Diamond realized that the indicator muscles would grow stronger in response to "positive or negative emotional and intellectual stimuli, as well as physical stimuli."[5] Dr. Hawkins took this concept further when he began researching the "kinesiological response to truth and falsehood" in 1975.[6]

Comments I have received from my demonstration of kinesiology on my website and YouTube have indicated that some people assert kinesiology and muscle testing are not the same. My assessment is that the way in which the tests are conducted is different, but the results are the same. Here I will outline the process for kinesiology, which requires two people and uses the large muscles of the body. In appendix 8: Kinesiology Testing Steps, I have included the process for muscle testing, which is done by one person and uses the fingers.

This is a simple explanation of kinesiology. Begin with two people. One is the subject, and the other is the tester. Have the subject stand tall, with one arm raised straight out from the side of the body and parallel to the floor. (There are variations on how to do this. You can use another large muscle, such as the leg, and you can also be sitting; however, in staying focused on Hawkins's study, our example will use the arm and have the person standing.) If it is the subject's left arm that is extended, then the tester faces the subject and places his or her left hand on the subject's right shoulder. It is suggested that the subject not look directly at the tester, but rather over the tester's shoulder. The tester then places her or his right hand on the subject's left wrist, with his or her palm facing downward. The tester can instruct the subject to resist when the tester pushes down on the wrist. Then the tester pushes down firmly on the wrist. The idea is to see whether the response is strong or weak, and there should be a bounce. It is not good for the tester to push too hard or for the subject to strain to resist, as this will fatigue the arm. Different people have different amounts of bounce in their arm as they are tested. Over time, the tester will know their testing answer—yes or no— quickly.

When you begin the kinesiology, the first question to ask should be a *yes* or *no* question or statement to ensure information is being received correctly. If you are the subject, an example would be for you to say, "My name is [your name]." When you test, you would get a *yes* response by your arm being strong while the tester pushes on it. Your next statement might be, "My name is Minnie Mouse." In this case, you would get a *no* response, meaning the arm the tester is pushing would be weak. To see if you are going to get an accurate response to subsequent questions, you should test strong for what is true and weak for what is false in this initial set, as it is a very simple example in which you know the answers.

If you are getting the wrong responses, then you are not communicating with yourself accurately. In this case, there are a couple of things you can do. One is to have a large glass of water. You may be dehydrated. The other would be a cross crawl. The cross crawl is an energy technique taught by Donna Eden.[7] She explains that it "facilitates the crossover of energy between the brain's right and left hemispheres."[8] She adds that the technique helps you to "feel more balanced, think more clearly, improve your coordination, and harmonize your energies."[9] Eden explains the steps for this technique as follows:

1. While standing, lift your right arm and left leg simultaneously.

2. After you let them down, raise your left arm and right leg. If you are unable to do this because, for instance, you are confined to a wheelchair, simply lift your knees to the opposite elbows, or twist your upper torso so your arm passes over the midline of your body.

2. Repeat, this time exaggerating the lift of your leg and the swing of your arm across the midline to the opposite side of your body.

3. Continue in this exaggerated march for at least a minute, again breathing deeply in through your nose and out through your mouth.[10]

The following section may not be for everyone, but for those who are interested, I have included information on the Map of Consciousness developed by Dr. Hawkins. I highly encourage you to get his book for yourself.

Dr. Hawkins has taken the process I just outlined even further. He found that this "kinesiologic response reflects the human organism's capacity to differentiate not only positive from negative stimuli, but also anabolic (life-threatening) from catabolic (life-consuming), and, most dramatically, truth from falsity."[11] In a simple test, there is a positive muscle reaction to an obviously true statement and a weak muscle reaction in response to a false statement. As Hawkins puts it, "This technique provides, for the first time in human history, an objective basis for distinguishing truth from falsehood, which is totally verifiable across time with randomly selected, naïve test subjects."[12]

With this test, Hawkins found he could calibrate consciousness. He used an arbitrary logarithmic scale of whole numbers, "stratifying the relative power of levels of consciousness in all areas of human experience."[13] With this scale, he conducted a twenty-year study that involved millions of calibrations.[14] The test subjects were from varying "walks of life," were of differing ages ranging from young children to people in their nineties, and had differing personality types.[15] The subjects mentally "ranged from what the world calls 'normal' to severely ill psychiatric patients," as well as landing on a broad continuum in terms of physical health. Furthermore, the subjects, who were of various nationalities, ethnic backgrounds, and religions, "were tested in Canada, the United States, Mexico, and throughout South America, Northern Europe, and the Far East."[16] Subjects were tested individually and in groups by many different testers and groups of testers. In all cases, without exception, the results were identical and entirely reproducible, fulfilling the fundamental requirement of the scientific method: perfect experimental replicability.[17]

Dr. Hawkins developed a Map of Consciousness that ranges from "shame," which calibrates at 20, to "enlightenment," which calibrates at anywhere from 700 to 1,000.[18] If you are interested, you can read more about this in his book. Hawkins explains that this scale can be used to "evaluate companies, movies, individuals, or events in history; it can also be used to diagnose current life problems."[19] The procedure is used to "verify the truth or falsity of a declarative statement."[20] It is important to be impersonal during the procedure, and "for accurate results, both persons doing the kinesiologic testing must themselves calibrate at level 200 (integrity) or above, and the motivation should be integrous."[21] Hawkins explains the procedure further:

> Once a numeric scale is elicited calibrations can be arrived at by stating, "This item" (such as this book, organization, this person's motive, and so on) "is over 100," then "over 200," then "over 300," until a negative response is obtained. The calibration can then be refined: "Is it over 220? 225? 230?," and so on. Tester and testee can trade places, and the same results will be obtained.[22]

I have included this information because kinesiology is an incredible diagnostic tool, as well as one that is extremely useful in self-healing. Many integrative health practitioners use kinesiology, and you're able to use it personally in many ways. Once you learn the muscle testing, which you can do yourself, you will be able to adapt this tool to your lifestyle. When using kinesiology, it is important that each participant be neutral and free of agendas and expectations. When you use it on yourself for healing, be aware that you must also remain neutral with no intention or expectation. At times this can be difficult. For myself, when I realize I may have Ego involved in the outcome, I will ask someone else to help me. Of course, if the process is being applied in hopes of healing, expectation and intention will both be present.

A specific way in which you might want to use this tool is to test the level of life energy in the food you eat. Imagine a scale. For example, you may use percentages. Let's use the example of an apple. As soon as the apple is picked from the tree, it begins to lose its life energy. This life energy is what nourishes your body. When you choose an apple, test the apple for the level of life left in it. A level of 100% would be the highest level of life, and 0% the lowest. To apply muscle testing using your fingers, either take the apple in one hand or touch one of your hands against the apple and test, starting at 10%, 20%, and so on, and see how high the percentage gets before your fingers release, signifying a *no*. That will give you knowledge about the level of life the apple has retained. I try to find food that has at least 70% of life left. During the summer, your food generally will have higher life energy. Think about it: how much life do you suppose is available in a can of green beans? Try muscle testing it and see. If you need further information or instruction on this technique, you may want to check out the videos called "Kinesiology" on my website at (**http://www.Candess Campbell.com**).

I have been blessed in having this tool at my disposal at several key moments in my life. One time that stands out for me was several years ago when my family—my dog Friday, my cat Kayla, and I—got sick at the same time. Friday and I fared well and recovered, but Kayla had a more difficult time. One evening I decided to take her to the pet emergency center. A friend of mine was in town and staying with me, so we went together. The vet checked Kayla and said he wanted to run a set of tests to see what was wrong. Well, truthfully, I have been resistive to medical testing and procedures as a first response, so I asked him if he would work with me. I asked what he was looking for with respect to the test results. He explained to me what organs might be involved in Kayla's illness. My response was to muscle test, and my testing showed it was the stomach. Then I asked him, "If it's the stomach, what would the treatment be?" He gave me the names of a couple of medications he thought might be helpful in that circumstance. I muscle tested and picked a medication. Kayla was severely dehydrated, having been sick for a few days, and the vet kept her overnight.

The next day when we went to get her, the vet announced, "She's good!" We looked at him questioningly, and he responded that he had decided to run the test on his own, the results of which indicated that I had been right. The problem was with the stomach, and the medicine Kayla had muscle tested for was what he would have given her. I was delighted with this feedback and the ability to act as a bridge between traditional medicine and energy medicine. I shared with the vet about Reiki as well, which I touched on earlier in this book and will talk about more again in the last week.

Another example that surprised me took place when I awoke one morning and found something wrong with my neck. It was kinked, and my head was twisted to the left in an odd position. I was in so much pain that I could hardly move, and when I moved accidentally, it really hurt. I was frightened and didn't know what to do. I had neither medical insurance nor a regular medical doctor. Finally, I remembered my friend, who was a massage therapist.[23] I called him and asked if he could help me. He came right over with his massage table and intuitively asked me some specific questions that had to do with my beliefs. He used muscle testing as well.

As he began asking me questions, I had a strange image of a past lifetime. I saw that in the past lifetime, my husband was physically abusive to my (our) children. My response had been to look away; I didn't do anything to help them. Once I realized this as I lay on the massage table, I felt remorseful. Then the muscles in my neck loosened, and I was fine. I realized then that this image had been triggered by a John Grisham movie I viewed the previous evening, in which there was a similar scene. It appeared that my neck became stuck as I would not turn my head to look at what was happening to my children. The effect of Robert's kinesiology and his newly learned skill at asking just the right questions to get to the core of the issue turned out to be miraculous. Dreams can also cause this kind of situation, and the healing would be the same process. I am confident it was from a past life only because I have been taking clients through past life hypnotherapy for many years.

Acupuncture

Acupuncture is commonly used for pain management in the United States. To begin to understand the world of acupuncture, it is important to be aware of the differences in the Eastern and Western approaches to medicine. In ancient China, people believed the body was sacred. As such, they never cut into the body. Of course we now know the deficiencies that result from that kind of thought: people died without surgery. That being said, the Chinese were reluctant to engage in surgeries because they looked at the body as a landscape or garden. Medical diagnoses in China take the form of nature metaphors. For example, in the West, one may be diagnosed with asthma. According to Cheyenne Mendel, in China, a patient presenting with the same symptoms may be diagnosed as: "Kidney chi fails to grasp the lung chi," "Lung yin deficiency," or "Wood counteracts metal." Each of these three diagnoses would result in a prescription for a different herbal formula and configuration of acupuncture.

Back pain is another example. In the West, the primary allopathic treatment is the same for everyone—painkillers or surgery. Western medicine has a history of exploring the body in detail. It was dissected, looked at under a microscope, and subjected to various scientific tests and studies. The body was seen as a conglomeration of disparate parts. In fact, the first or second page of any anatomy textbook talks about the body as a machine. With a machine, if something is broken, you fix it. If it is bad, you replace it. If something is missing, you add to it. It is easy to see, given this mindset, how we have gotten to the point of being dependent on medications to treat various symptoms.

The good news is that we now have access to the healing methods of both Eastern and Western cultures. Calling holistic medicine "alternative medicine" is no longer appropriate. The best approach now is "integrated medicine," in which we take the best of both worlds. Remember, the concept of acupuncture was initially very hard for Western minds to grasp, because we didn't have the concept of *chi*. In the 1970s, George Lucas's *Star Wars* debuted, and the mass consciousness was introduced to the notion of "the force." Chi is life force energy.

If something is alive, it has chi. When the chi in your body is flowing, you have health. When it is blocked, you have stagnation of chi, or disease (dis-ease). The organ in Chinese medicine that is believed to be responsible for moving chi is the liver. What we would diagnose as depression in the West would be considered liver chi stagnation in the East. Many times, when pain is present, the chi is simply stuck. Inserting a few needles moves the chi, and the pain goes away. If a person is depressed and prescribed medication, the drug can put even more stress on a stagnant liver. This is an issue as the liver is the detox organ that helps process these drugs.

Acupuncture is not mysterious. The body heals itself, plain and simple. It is an electrical system. Inserting tiny metal filaments at certain points in the body helps the body heal itself faster, by moving the chi.

Acupuncture is used often for pain and to help those who are addicted to drugs. Inserting acupuncture needles in the ears has been shown to help people detox from drugs. The ear is a micro system; the whole body can be mapped on the ear. Most people have heard of foot reflexology. All organs, the skeleton, the brain, the limbs, the entire body can be mapped on the feet. The ear is also a body map. Because the ear is so close to the brain, putting needles in the ear stimulates endorphin release. Endorphins are opiate-like.

When a person has had pain for a long time, that individual's tolerance increases. If he or she has taken painkillers for some time, the medication is not as effective as it was originally. The brain no longer manufactures the same level of natural opiate, because there is a regular external supply coming in. If the person stops taking the medication, the brain does not automatically kick in right away and produce natural painkillers. However, according to acupuncturist Cheyenne Mendel, acupuncture can provide that function instantaneously. Often people feel very "high" right after receiving treatment, due to the endorphin release. That high levels off as the body comes into balance after a few acupuncture treatments.

To further understand acupuncture, it is important to start with the meridian system. In Chinese medicine, the meridian system is seen as an energetic system deep within the tissues of the body. There are twelve meridians that correlate to the organs of the body. The acupuncturist will diagnose what treatment is needed based partially on the twelve pulses. Each pulse is related to one of the meridians. The meridians are the energetic system through which the chi, or life force, runs. There are specific acupuncture points along the meridians that are known to relate directly to the organs. In Chinese medicine, the intent of the treatment is to support the body's coming into balance. As we explore other energy medicine tools for self-healing, it is important to understand that the meridians are the map for the acupuncture points and the healing points. There are many sources online and in bookstores that will help you to see where the meridians are in the body.

Donna Eden's 1999 book, *Energy Medicine*, is a great resource for self-healing.[24] She explains that you can balance your meridians and get them flowing correctly to increase your health by (1) tracing your meridians with your finger, (2) flushing congested meridians by movement of the hands over the meridian in a specific manner, (3) twisting and stretching in ways that affect particular meridians, (4) massaging "the meridian's neurolymphatic points," and (5) tapping or holding specific acupuncture points that are located on the meridian.[25]

Eden's groundbreaking work has been helpful to many, and I include myself on that list. This one resource is invaluable. You may find practitioners in your area who either use Eden's techniques or teach her work. Later in this week's material I will share some simple exercises of hers that can make a big difference in your energy level and your health.

It is common for pain to diminish when the energy that was congested becomes freed. According the U.S. National Institute of Health, "Acupuncture is being studied for its efficacy in alleviating many kinds of pain. There are promising findings in some conditions, such as chronic low-back pain and osteoarthritis of the knee; but, for most other conditions, additional research is needed. The National Center for Complementary and Alternative Medicine (NCCAM) sponsors a wide range of acupuncture research."[26]

Some other energy medicine tools we will learn about when focusing on self-healing include flower essences, essential oils, crystals, and gem elixirs. I have listed some resources where you can find these products and more information on them in appendix 9: Trauma and Healing Resources.

Flower Essences

In his book, *Vibrational Medicine*, Richard Gerber, MD gives several examples of how our subtle energy bodies are affected by other energies. He explains:

> Our subtle-energy bodies play a major role in maintaining our health. Energy disturbances in the etheric body precede the manifestation of abnormal patterns of cellular organization and growth. Disease becomes manifest in the physical body only after disturbances of energy flow have already become crystallized in the subtle structural patterns of the higher frequency bodies.[27]

In the chakra section, we talked about the subtle energy bodies and how they are related to health. Vibrational medicines each have a different frequency, and Gerber suggests using high-frequency vibrational medicines to alter the dysfunctional patterns in your body. *Frequency* is the same as *vibration*, and the way I like to explain it is that everything vibrates at a different rate. For instance, imagine that ice vibrates at a lower level (or frequency) than water. Water vibrates at a lower frequency than mist. The vibration rate determines the density of matter. Gerber describes subtle matter as vibrating at a speed that exceeds that of the velocity of light. Vibrational medicines such as essences or tinctures each have their own particular vibration and can be used for different health purposes.

The most well-known flower essence remedies were developed by Dr. Edward Bach of England.[28] Gerber explains that Bach was a traditional physician who had made bacteriology his specialty. Early on, Bach noticed that particular bacteria were found in the gastrointestinal tracts of patients who had chronic illnesses. He isolated these bacteria and noted their presence in patients suffering from such ailments as rheumatic disorders and arthritis. Bach calculated that increasing the patients' immune response relative to those particular microorganisms might result in their experiencing fewer symptoms. He therefore concocted vaccines made from those very intestinal bacteria. "When given by injection to patients with various chronic disorders," Gerber reports, "the vaccines produced significant improvements in the arthritic and other chronic symptoms."[29]

Gerber also notes that Bach later was given Samuel Hahnemann's book, *The Organon of Medicine*, which introduced him to the concept of homeopathy. Through experimenting over time, Gerber relates, Bach "classified seven types of bacteria associated with chronic illness" that became known as Bach's Seven Nosodes. In the process, Bach noticed that patients with these seven types of intestinal bacteria pathogens "displayed particular personality types or temperaments."[30] This was the beginning of Bach's understanding of the emotional and mental connection to physical illness, as he found the following:

> [P]atients in the same personality group would react to their illnesses in a similar fashion with the same behaviors, moods, and states of mind, regardless of the disease. Therefore, it was necessary only to categorize the mental and emotional characteristics of the patient in order to find which remedy would be most applicable to curing their chronic illness.[31]

Gerber points out, "What Bach had correctly intuited was that different emotional and personality factors contribute toward a general predisposition to illness. The most significant of these factors were emotional tendencies such as fear and negative attitudes." Gerber adds that Bach had come to this conclusion over half a century before the advent of modern-day psychoneuroimmunological research.[32]

According to Gerber, Bach had figured out that the "illness-personality link was an outgrowth of dysfunctional energetic pattern within the subtle bodies" and believed that "illness was a reflection of disharmony between the physical personality and the Higher Self or soul."[33] Thus, Bach sought to find natural elements that, rather than treating an established disease, would deal with the emotional states that tend to herald the onset of disease.[34] He developed a total of thirty-eight essences, including his last, which was a combination of floral mixtures called Rescue Remedy.[35]

Because my beliefs about self-healing are so much in alignment with Bach's writing, and because my intent is to bridge traditional healing and spiritual healing, I am strongly drawn to Bach's work. Gerber cites Bach as having explained that every human is incarnated to learn and grow—to figure out and manifest his or her purpose—and that until that happens, each person experiences a struggle between his or her soul and personality, which results in physical illness.[36]

As a psychic "sensitive," Bach was able to discover how the flowers worked through his own observation of how they affected him.[37] Like many psychics and sensitives, myself included, he found the "bustling crowds and chaos ... too disruptive and draining."[38] Bach lived in the English countryside and, after falling prey to an illness that nearly took his life, turned to nature to find healing. Gerber reports that Bach found his sensitivity was such that he could

> touch the morning dew from a flower or its petal to his lips and he would experience the potential therapeutic effects of the plant. Bach was so sensitive when he was exposed to a particular flower, he would experience all of the physical symptoms and emotional states to which the flower's essence was an antidote. This was such a strain on him physically and emotionally that he died in 1936 at age 56.[39]

Flower essences continued to be prepared by the Dr. Edward Bach Healing Centre after his death, and new essences have been developed.[40]

Much experimentation continued in the study of flower essences, and Richard Katz established the Flower Essence Society in 1979. This group provided a framework for therapists and flower essence workers to network and exchange information. Katz was also able to get clinical feedback about the success or failure of the essences. According to Gerber, this feedback "indicated that the new essences worked especially well with the process of inner growth and spiritual awakening."[41]

Although Bach developed the remedies that affected the emotional body to prevent illness, it was Gurudas who categorized flower essences into two groups. One works primarily with the physical body, and the other at the level of the subtle bodies, chakras, and various psychological states. The Bach Remedies would fit more closely with the second group.[42]

Gurudas' 1986 book, *Flower Essences and Vibrational Healing*, describes 108 new flower essences.[43] Gerber notes, "The author's description of the effects of the essences upon the human body contains extremely technical biochemical and energetic information about their mechanisms of action."[44] Gurudas' information came through Kevin Ryerson, a channeling source similar in ability to Edgar Cayce.[45] A channeler is one who goes into a meditative or trance-like state to receive information from a spiritual guide or a spiritual source. Gerber explains that Ryerson both describes the effects of the various essences and gives vital information concerning the subtle workings of the human body.[46]

One of the flower essences that the Flower Essence Society claims is helpful for chronic pain is impatiens. On its website **(http://www.flowersociety.org/impatiens-cases .htm)**, the Flower Essence Society also provides a downloadable copy of Patricia Kaminski's *Choosing Flower Essence*, which describes how to choose the correct essence based on some experiences you have had or ways in which you experience the world.[47] I noticed the Flower Essence Society had specific trauma and illness questions related to the herb *arnica*. Years ago, when my poodle Friday was diagnosed with colitis, the veterinarian gave me arnica as a remedy, and it was helpful. Information found on the website listed at the start of this paragraph may be helpful in finding the flower essence(s) that may benefit you. It may also give you some insight into your personality and how you experience your life.

This topic brings to mind my experience in wandering through a mall in Tokyo after facilitating a workshop. Feeling really stressed after such a busy schedule, I was seeking some help. I saw a kiosk with Bach Flower Remedies, and although I had used essential oils before, I did not have much experience with flower essences. After muscle testing the remedies (a concept I reference numerous times in this book) to see which would be helpful, I noted testing strong for vervain. As soon as I put a few drops under my tongue, I could feel the stress just fall from my body, especially down my back. I took a deep breath and felt as if I had just released an incredible amount of stress. When I got home, I looked up vervain on the Bach website and found the following description, written by Dr. Bach:

> Those with fixed principles and ideas, which they are confident are right, and which they very rarely change. They have a great wish to convert all around them to their own views of life. They are strong of will and have much courage when they are convinced of those things that they wish to teach. In illness they struggle on long after many would have given up their duties.[48]

I can see how this helped me relax after publicly facilitating a workshop and presenting a public face, what I refer to as "being on." I was delighted to have found this remedy and so happy to have the tool of muscle testing to choose the essence that was right for me.

I had a related experience during a session with my psychiatrist friend, who is also a shaman and acupuncturist. He suggested I get some angelica, which is another essence.

I did as he suggested. Later, I found angelica oil helps relax nerves and muscles. It also restores happy memories and helps with peaceful sleep. Although I am not sure what he was seeing while reading me, this was another instance in which energy medicine helped me tremendously. Afterward, I felt grounded, connected to myself, and better able to relate to others.

Essential Oils

In addition to flower essences, there are essential oils. You already understand that everything has a vibration and that one of the goals in healing is to become balanced and raise your vibration. Emotional and physical stress disrupt this balance. The stress then blocks the flow of life energy, and the result is inflammation, irritation, and illness.[49] While pharmaceutical drugs have no life force and cause side effects, the vibratory quality of plants assists in bringing the body into harmony. It does so through oil molecules that resonate with the frequencies needed for the body.[50] In an aromatherapy class I attended, author Linda Smith explained that science has understood the healing properties of plants and has indeed made medicines with them. I also learned that essential oils can assist in healing toxins and negative emotions in your body. This is because the oils don't resonate with the toxins and negative emotions.

In his 1998 book, *Freedom Through Health*, Dr. Terry Shepherd Friedmann tells us that healing is the body's movement toward an active state of balance.[51] He expresses the belief that we are always moving toward a state of healthy equilibrium, and that a healer's work is to be of assistance in that process. Friedmann adds that disease may look like (and in fact result in) chemical imbalance, but he explains that the chemical imbalance proceeds from an electromagnetic imbalance that has changed the body at a fundamental level. By providing the appropriate frequency to bring cells back to balance, healers can help people to increase their health. Raising someone's vibration, Friedmann asserts, results in restored physical health, mental clarity, and spiritual attunement.[52] This is the work of essential oils.

The frequencies of essential oils range from 52 to 320 megahertz.[53] Each oil has its own frequency that will have an effect on your subtle energy field. Some examples of the frequencies of oils are listed here.

Rose (*Rosa damascene*) .... 320 MHz

Lavender (*Lavendula angustifola*) .... 118 MHz

Myrrh *(Commihora myrrha)* .... 105 MHz

Blue Chamomile *(Matricaria recutita)* ...... 105 MHz

Juniper *(Juniperus osteosperma)* .... 98 MHz

Aloes/Sandalwood (*Santalum album*) .... 96 MHz

Angelica *(Angelica archanelica)* .... 85 MHz

Peppermint (*Mentha peperita*) .... 78 MHz

Galbanum *(Ferula Gummosa)* .... 56 MHz

Basil *(Ocimum basilicum)* .... 52 MHz

Smith notes that unadulterated essential oils have strong frequencies, whereas those that are not pure may have frequencies that drop to 0 MHz.[54] She asserts that when a person breathes in an essential oil, there can be a sudden shift in that person's frequency—higher if the oil is pure, lower if it is not. Smith adds that the environment created by essential oils is not hospitable to viruses, harmful bacteria, fungal disease, and similar elements; in fact, she claims that these detrimental elements cannot survive in the presence of pure essential oils.[55]

As you read through this information, bear in mind that you can use the essential oil, flower essence, or plant essence for the same issue. For instance, if you want to become more grounded—more connected to the earth—with more of your attention in present time, you can get the essential oil called Grounding by Young Living Essential Oils, or you can use the same essences in plant essence form.[56]

The following information on essential oils as they relate to the chakras is taken from Salvatore Battaglia's 2003 book, *The Complete Guide to Aromatherapy*.[57] The information in reference to the Young Living Essential Oils comes from the Young Living website at **http://cc.younglivingworld.com**.

Essential Oils for the Chakras

Essential oils are natural and can be helpful for the issues outlined in the chakras section in Week Ten. Once you have identified the issues, you can use muscle testing or the following information to determine essential oils you may want to use. Please note, you are in charge of your health and are responsible for the choices you make, including whether or not you choose these oils. Throughout this book, you will find my belief in the importance of using both allopathic and integrative medicine.

Chakra One – The Base and First Chakra

There are several essential oils that resonate well with the first chakra. The issues of the first chakra have to do with your roots—feeling grounded and nourished, as well as safe and connected to your family and your tribe. I use the following Young Living Essential Oils: Grounding, Present Time, and Longevity. Others that resonate with the first chakra are vetiver, angelica, patchouli, or tree essential oils such as juniper, cedar wood, pine, spruce and fir. These essential oils are all generally grounding, centering, and strengthening.

Chakra Two – The Sacral and Second chakra

The issues of the second chakra deal with relationships, emotions, intimacy, sexuality, creativity, work, and money. The oils I generally use for the second chakra are the following, by Young Living: Magnify Your Purpose and Inner Child. Young Living recommends Dragon Time for premenstrual syndrome (PMS). Individual essential oils that resonate with the second chakra include sandalwood, patchouli, jasmine, and rose. They connect with the sexual energy and are warming and sensual.

Chakra Three – The Solar and Third chakra

The issues in the third chakra relate to vitality, as well your energy level, inner strength, power, control, identity, and self-esteem. The Young Living Essential Oils I use for the third chakra are En-R-Gee, Juniper, Vetiver, and Peppermint. En-R-Gee helps with circulation and vitality. Juniper is a cleanser and detoxifier. Vetiver is grounding and stabilizing; it is also helpful for stress and dealing with trauma. Peppermint is helpful for soothing digestion and has been researched for positive effects on the liver and respiratory system by Jean Valnet, MD.[58] It has also been studied for its role in increasing one's ability to smell or taste after their senses have been impaired. I shared earlier that I lost my sense of smell in an accident when I was fourteen years old. Even though this is so, I have only and always been able to smell peppermint when it was in steam (such as tea). Peppermint has also been studied for its ability to improve concentration and mental accuracy.

Chakra Four – The Heart and Fourth Chakra

The issues in the fourth chakra deal with love of self, love of others, and love of the God of your heart, as well as forgiveness, compassion, hope, and trust. The essential oils I use for this chakra are Young Living's Believe and Inner Child. Believe (the essential oil just mentioned) was designed to open you to your highest beliefs. You can also use rose, ylang ylang, and neroli. The other Young Living Essential Oil mentioned in this section, Inner Child, is developed to bring emotional balance. As it helps with identity as well, it is a good choice for the third chakra. Rose brings balance and harmony. According to Young Living, ylang ylang is a symbol of love. The pale yellow petals are fragrant and often strewn across the marriage bed. It has a softer floral scent and is often used instead of the sweeter rose. Neroli was an essential oil used in Egypt and is known to have healing properties.

Chakra Five – The Throat and Fifth Chakra

The issues in the fifth chakra relate to communication, choice, will, decision-making, needs, and self-expression. I like to use Gathering from Young Living, an essential oil created to help overcome the chaotic energy that interferes with focus. When communicating, this is very helpful. The blend used in this Young Living essential oil helps in gathering your emotional and spiritual thoughts. It contains galbanum, a favorite oil of Moses. In addition to galbanum, the mix includes frankincense, sandalwood, lavender, cinnamon, rose, spruce, geranium, and ylang ylang, which makes it a great starter oil.

Battaglia says German chamomile and Roman chamomile both impart calm strength and enable the truth to be spoken without anger.[59] These oils resonate with the throat chakra and encourage the expression of spiritual truth. Of course, you can also use Young Living's Chamomile (and some others that are pure) as a tea to help you relax in the evening.

Chakra Six – The Third Eye and Sixth Chakra

The information contained in the sixth chakra relates to insight, clairvoyance, intuition, self-evaluation, intellect, and wisdom. My favorite essential oils for the sixth chakra are Young Living's Brain Power and Clarity. Brain Power is a specially designed blend of oils high in sesquiterpenes, a defensive agent that crosses the blood-brain barrier. It is used to clarify and support concentration. Clarity is also used to assist in mental alertness. According to Young Living, rosemary and peppermint are in this blend and have been used for years for mental activity and vitality.[60] They state that at the University of Cincinnati, Dr. William N. Dember discovered in a research study that inhaling peppermint oil increased the mental accuracy of the students he tested by twenty-eight percent. Young Living's Everlasting essential oil activates the right side of the brain, deepening intuition and facilitating access to the unconsciousness, while Thyme essential oil stimulates the left brain and all conscious and intellectual thoughts.[61]

Juniper berry, rosemary, thyme and basil—when used with appropriate visualization—help to connect with the higher levels of the mind and bring clarity to our understanding of spiritual truths.

Chakra Seven – The Crown and Seventh Chakra

The seventh chakra relates to what you know, as well as your values and ethics, courage, selflessness, inspiration, spirituality, and devotion. I usually use Envision by Young Living for this chakra. Envision is a blend of essential oils that help bring renewed faith in the future and maintain the emotional fortitude necessary to achieve your goals and dreams.

Battaglia explains that French Alpine lavender, rosewood, sandalwood, frankincense, and myrrh are wonderful oils to use with the crown chakra. Rosewood facilitates the opening of the crown chakra, and frankincense has the ability to connect us with the Divine within and without.[62]

There are essential oils that are known to be helpful for pain as well. You can use specific oils depending upon the situation. Pain can come from everyday aches, bone pain, chronic pain, pain in the joints, muscle pain, surgical pain, or tissue pain. There are several resources that will help you determine which oils will be best for you. You will see that many of the chakras above list the same oils, so you may want to start your collection with oils that can help more than one at a time. A book I recommend for learning more about essential oils is Connie and Alan Quigley's, entitled *Quick Reference Guide for Using Essential Oils.*[63]

Some essential oils are used *neat,* which means they are placed directly on the skin. Others must be put in a carrier oil such as almond or sunflower oil. Young Living's Pan-Away contains wintergreen, which needs a carrier oil. You can rub it on your temples, the back of your neck, your forehead, or the bottom of your feet. You can also inhale this oil. I have used this particular one several times, usually for lower back pain. In rubbing it on my lower back, the pain subsides quickly. Using a carrier oil can also extend the time the essential oil stays in your energy field.

I hope this was a helpful introduction to using essential oils for your health. As treatment modalities go, this one is fun and smells good too!

Crystals

Another form of energy medicine is the use of crystals. Although a number of people cannot access detailed information from higher frequencies, those with clairvoyant ability are able to do so. Many have seen and experienced the healing properties of crystals. From Gerber's writings, it appears that science is beginning to catch up with this ancient knowledge. We are starting to see the importance of crystals and the extent to which we've been unaware of their significant properties. In this section, I will address the healing properties of high vibration crystals.

One of the most common crystals used by healers is the quartz. Gerber cites Miller's 1984 interview with Marcel Vogel, who was a senior scientist with IBM for twenty-seven years, as well as a crystal researcher. Vogel is quoted as saying that the crystal is a neutral object whose inner structure exhibits a state of perfection and balance. When it's cut to the proper form, and when the human mind enters into relationship with its structural perfection, the crystal emits a vibration that extends and amplifies the powers of the user's mind. Like a laser, it radiates energy in a coherent, highly concentrated form, and this energy may be transmitted to objects or people at will.[64]

Gerber reports Vogel further explaining that although the crystal can be used for telepathic purposes, its loftier purpose is alleviating human suffering. Vogel added that a properly trained healer uses crystals to help people let go of negative thoughtforms that have manifested as illness in a patient's body.[65] A thoughtform is defined by Gerber as "a manifestation of a strong thought or emotion as an actual energetic structure within an individual's auric field."[66] According to the thoughts expressed here by Vogel, thoughtforms have a distinct effect on a person's health and can be eliminated, if necessary, through the use of crystals.

Each stone or gem has different properties—even those within the same family. On my website (**http://www.12 WeeksToSelfHealing.com**) you will find an interview with Charles Lightwalker, an intuitive shaman who wrote the *Crystal and Stone Healing Home Study Course*.[67] If you find you are interested in crystals, you may want to find a book on them or learn through his class. You can learn which crystals are best for healing a particular issue, as well as how to choose and care for them. For example, it is a common practice to put your crystals in the sunlight occasionally to clear them. Some crystals will increase and some will absorb, so be sure to research carefully in order to use them most advantageously. While I provide an introduction to crystals in this week, I hope you will continue to explore on your own.

Lightwalker encourages his students to go to a gem shop and experience the crystals and stones. He advises you will be drawn to the ones that are best for you, saying that it is "the stone calling you"—trust your intuition in finding the right crystals and stones.

As an introduction to crystals and how they relate to other concepts within this book, I would like to share with you some helpful tips on those that are related to the chakras.

For the first chakra, I would start with a set of quartz crystals. Like many other crystals, quartz crystals provide healing, energizing, and access to higher dimensions.[68] Clear quartz is one of the most popular of the quartz stones. These crystals also magnify the power of other stones. They are usually readily available in many sizes.

For the second or sacral chakra, you may want to choose a cubic crystal, such as a garnet or fluorite; these stones resonate with the issues of the sacral chakra. A diamond does as well, but it may be too expensive. The cubic crystals have a building block energy pattern and can be used with fundamental issues, with meditation, or when dealing with basic issues of everyday life. They assist in the repair of damaged cellular structures, from the DNA up to the skeletal system.[69]

Next, for the third or solar chakra, you may want to choose an aquamarine. This crystal is of the hexagonal classification, which also includes emeralds and apatite. These stones encourage growth and vitality, balance energy, and are good for communicating and storing information. They are useful when you want to move into service to others.[70] When you are in pain, you may find yourself isolating, and this stone can be helpful in getting you out into the open and focused outside of yourself. Once you get out, you are often happy that you did. This might be because you are able to match other people's energy and lift your vibration, especially if you are doing something you enjoy, like helping others.

For the fourth or heart chakra, you may want to try wulfenite from the Red Cloud mine in Arizona. This stone belongs to the tetragonal system, as do zircon and chalcopyrite. Interestingly, wulfenite balances by absorbing negativity, transmuting it, and giving back a positive vibration. It channels energies between the earth and higher dimensions.[71] This conversion is especially helpful when you are lonely or grieving.

The fifth chakra, which is the throat chakra, is connected to the orthorhombic system, and stones helpful in clearing this chakra include the peridot, topaz, and alexandrite. They have a pattern of "encircling and encompassing energy patterns, problems, and thought forms."[72] They tend to bring perspective to situations and to magnify and clear what is irrelevant! These stones help individuals isolate problems and contain them until the issues can be worked out. As stated throughout this book, it is important to get to the root of problems so they can be released.

The stones for the sixth chakra, also knows as the third eye chakra, are malachite, azurite, jade, and moonstone. These stones are in the monoclinic system and have a constant pulsing action. They continually expand and contract, which creates a movement into action, growth, and increased consciousness. They tend to clear our paths by dissolving problems and moving us into a higher consciousness.[73] Recently, when I was in Victoria, British Columbia, I saw a jade sculpture that was about four feet in height and eighteen inches wide. It had eagles carved from jade attached at the top and salmon near the bottom. The energy around this beautiful sculpture was so amazing that it was difficult for me to leave the shop. Simply being in the presence of these stones is healing.

For the seventh or crown chakra, you may want to find a beautiful turquoise or rhodonite. These stones belong to the triclinic system. Triclinic crystals tend to promote totality or completeness. They help to balance the yin and yang energy within an individual.[74] The yin and the yang are universal opposites that can oppose each other, balance each other, or reverse from one to the other. Gerber explains that they aid in merging and harmonizing polarities that are unbalanced, which can include personalities.[75] This kind of treatment is good for extreme attitudes that may create discord.

You also may want to experience gems in the trigonal system. Being an Aquarian, I love amethyst and wear it often. You may find, as a result of wearing amethyst, that your energy can be transmuted to a higher level and that negative energies can be repelled. Amethyst amplifies the healing energy that affects your subtle body in a positive way. Gerber notes that it has a high vibratory rate, is associated with the ultraviolet spectrum, and may even help with cellular replication. Amethyst helps the flow of the life force and is able to affect blood vessels and arteries by carrying this energy through the bloodstream, meaning it works as a purifier. Amethyst works in the etheric field more than on a specific chakra, although it can be used for specific areas of the body. For example, by putting it over a blood clot, you can help dissolve the clot. Wherever it is used, it is able to help the blood flow become re-energized and move more freely.[76]

Carnelians, agates, and bloodstones are also gems in the trigonal system. They all help to balance your subtle energy body. They can be helpful in bringing you back into balance when you experience a lack of energy. Additionally, they help to balance the brain, thereby assisting with clarity.

When you have had some experience with stones and gems, you will know what your body responds to best. Lightwalker recommends starting with hematite for grounding. He also says that our own birthstone is a good one with which to begin. And remember that this is just an overview. If you are interested in working with crystals, you will find they are extremely helpful in self-healing and are fascinating as well. When working with crystals, be sure to do research, as some of the gems and stones will either increase or decrease energies, and it is important that you are aware of how you are affecting your subtle energy bodies. Starting with quartz crystals is both safe and healing.

Protection

Most of us who are in need of healing tend to be particularly sensitive to others' energy, but all of us are affected by the energy around us. When you feel good, you are running your own energy through your system. When you are feeling good and suddenly you don't feel well, there is a strong possibility that someone else has sent you some negative energy or a negative thought.

It is helpful to learn to protect yourself from others' energy. Although I do teach how to clear others' energy from your energy field, this week focuses on preventing yourself from being attacked energetically. You can do this through several techniques. Try different methods and find the ones that work best for you.

One way to protect yourself is with golden white light. Sit and imagine a golden white light in your heart. See this light expanding throughout your body and then expanding 6–8 inches beyond your body. Around this light, imagine a violet light extending about 12 inches. The golden white light is protective, but it may be too bright for some as they look at you. The violet light dims the brightness so that when others look at you, the image is calm and peaceful.

Another way to protect yourself is to imagine a golden white light coming down from the heavens through your crown chakra at the top of your head. This is Divine light. See the light filling your body and then expanding 6–8 inches beyond your body. Around this light, imagine a violet light extending about 12 inches.

Donna Eden has a technique called "zipping up." She asserts, "When you are feeling sad or vulnerable, the central meridian, the energy pathway that governs your central nervous system, can be like a radio receiver that channels other people's negative thoughts and energies into you. It's as if you are open and exposed."[77] You can use the subtle energy of your hand to zip up the central meridian, which runs like a zipper from your pubic bone up to your bottom lip. When you zip up, Eden explains, you will "feel more confident and positive about your world, think more clearly, tap inner strengths, and protect yourself from negative energies that may be around you."[78]

To zip up, you will tap K-27 acupuncture points. You can find them by placing

> your fingers on your collarbone (clavicle). Now slide them inward toward the center and find the bumps where they stop. Drop about an inch beneath these corners and slightly outward to the K-27s. Most people have a slight indent here that their fingers will drop into.[79]

Next, Eden recommends that you place your hand at the pubic bone. I like to have people imagine they have a jacket on and that the zipper starts at the pubic bone or first chakra. Eden suggests that you take a deep breath while moving your hand up, as if you were zipping up the jacket to your bottom lip, and then turn as if you are locking a key. Do this three times. Next, imagine as if you have on a hood. Take your hand to the back of your neck where the hood may connect to your shirt. Zip up over the top of your head straight down to the top of your lip, and turn as if you are turning a lock (in either direction). Eden advises you to do this three times as well.[80]

This technique can be done several times a day. You can pair it with using the restroom in washing your hands, zipping up, and leaving. This technique is especially helpful when you work where there are a lot of people or with people who are angry, stressed, or ill.

If you were to have someone test you with kinesiology, you would find yourself testing strong having done this. There are times when someone may "look you down." This can take away your strength, and you would test weak. Also, people can throw negative energy or thoughts at you, resulting in your testing weak. By using this zipping up technique, you stay strong. I remember watching a video of

Donna Eden's, *Energy Healing*, years ago. She had someone from the audience come up in front of the group. This person tested weak, and she subsequently had him read to the audience. Then she tested the people in the front row, and they all tested weak. After having the man zip up, he tested strong. He read to the audience again, and she tested the people in the front row once more. This time, they too tested strong. What this showed is that we match those we are around, especially those who are influencing us or instructing us. I think of our teachers in the school system and how powerful it would be if they knew this and could strengthen themselves, thereby strengthening their students.

When I was working as a mental health counselor at the Healing Lodge of the Seven Nations in Spokane, Washington, I worked with primarily Native American adolescents who were recovering from alcohol and drugs. I loved working with these young men and women, but given that they were struggling with figuring out their lives in a residential treatment program as well as managing their bodies' changes and roaring hormones, I definitely zipped up many times a day.

I also remember having a client who was an international musician. During her performance in downtown Spokane, she said she got out on stage and found she didn't feel very good energetically. She thought for a moment and decided to zip up right there on stage. Afterward, she said she sang better than she had in a long time. I was so proud of her.

Another great energy medicine tool from Eden is to walk backwards. I don't remember now where I learned this incredible tool, but I believe it was at a workshop where another healer was using Eden's techniques. When you find you are moving too fast, doing too much, and always in a rush, it helps to walk backwards. The energy within our body gets moving, and we are energetically ahead of ourselves. By walking backward and then forward, we somehow get back within ourselves energetically. Try it—this really helps!

Experiment with the list below and find what works best for you. It is helpful to use your journal and rate your pain on the pain scale first, and then use one tool at a time to see how you are able to change the pain level. Keep track of this in your journal. You may also want to find a friend who will support you in this. As you talk about your progress and your friend or other supportive person asks you questions, you are likely to stay on track and continue with your self-healing plan.

Tools and Exercises

1. Write down some declarative statements, one per paper, to practice kinesiology. Fold the paper so you do not know what each paper says. Find a friend and practice kinesiology. Hold the paper near your solar plexus (in front of your body under your heart), while your friend tests your non-dominant arm. You may want to test movies, politicians, or medical providers in your life.

2. Learn muscle testing from the demonstrations in appendix 8: Kinesiology Testing Steps and/or watch my video demonstration at **http://www.CandessCampbell.com**.

3. Go to the grocery store and test the food you pick. Use a percentage scale. You will be surprised at

the difference from one piece of fruit to the next. Be sure to allow yourself to test without getting your Ego or head involved, because it is important to be in a neutral state. In addition to testing foods to determine the general level of life force in them, you can test food to see whether a particular food is likely to support your body. Think of the food, or hold it, and say the following to yourself, either silently or out loud: "This food, [whatever it is], will support my body and my health." You will get a strong response or a weak one. The response will tell you whether it is wise for you to have the food at that time. I almost always use this technique when I want to have a cup of coffee, ice cream, or a glass of wine. These are foods that my body will accept at some times and not at others. There is also a video on my website that teaches how to muscle test food.

4. Look through the information on chakras and see where you are out of balance. Choose a flower essence or an essential oil that will help you. Use muscle testing to see which is best for you. You can do this by just thinking about the flower essence or essential oil and then testing whether you are strong or weak. If you are strong for more than one, use a percentage scale. For instance, test one oil starting at 10%, then 20%, up to when the test breaks.

5. Purchase essential oils like lavender. Sit and breathe in a Divine breath. Put a drop of lavender essential oil in your palm and rub your hands

together. Bring your hands up to your face and breathe in the fragrance. Sit and relax for a few minutes, noticing any changes in your body and your emotions. Write for a few moments in your journal about what you experience. To help you sleep at night, you can put lavender on your pillow or on the bottom of your feet.

6. Find a quartz stone that feels right to you. You can use this crystal in different ways. You may want to put it by your bed when you sleep, carry it in your pocket, or put it in your bath while you relax and receive the energy.

7. Practice zipping up daily. Notice the difference it makes in your energy throughout the day. Teach your friends and family to zip up as well.

8. Practice walking backwards when you are pushing yourself too hard. See if you feel better at the end of the day.

9. Practice breathing fear, anger, and pain *out* of your lungs and body. Imagine smelling a rose as you breathe in, and imagine blowing out a candle as you breathe out.[81] This is quite effective. Use a pain scale to notice the difference.

10. When you feel pain, put your hands on the area that hurts. You naturally have healing energy in your hands. Rub your hands together first to feel the healing energy in your hands. You can also rub and stretch the area. Using an essential oil here would be helpful as well.

11. Invest in a book that teaches you about the acupuncture points and how to hold them yourself. Practice this technique. I recommend Michael Reed Gach's book, *Acu-Yoga: Self Help Techniques to Relieve Tension.*[82]

12. Take your journal and write what you learned about yourself while reading the information on energy medicine. What did you already know at some level, and what is totally new to you? What will you incorporate into your life after having read this week? Journal about what has been helpful for you.

Week Twelve: Integrate and Receive

Where Does My Energy Go?

Do you notice you are tired in the morning when you first awake? Do you have a difficult time concentrating? Where does your energy go? I love the work of Caroline Myss—especially her image of the hundred circuits of energy we are given each day. In a course called Medical Intuition Training that she taught in April of 2004, she described these energy circuits as your power or your Spirit. She had us imagine one hundred circuits coming out from the top of our heads. She then asked us to follow the circuits to see where they were going. We imagined that 20% of the circuits were in the future, as people thought about what they were going to do later in the day; 40% in the past, connected to a childhood wound; and 30% in present time, leaving 10% unaccounted for.

When your energy is not in present time, you do not have the energy to fuel your body-mind. To be able to heal your body, you need to have a large percentage of your energy in present time. This explains partially why some people are able to heal themselves quickly and others are not. To bring your energy back, I have given you several tools of grounding and meditating. Utilizing self-hypnosis and receiving hypnosis from a professional will be helpful as well. The process of becoming conscious is inherent in all the tools and techniques presented in this book. Becoming conscious is necessary for self-healing. Your writings will be invaluable in learning to know yourself and love yourself.

Reassessing My Symptoms

By this time, you may have made several changes in your behavior, and it is time to assess how you are doing. Let's start by having you complete another Sensory Description of Pain sheet from Week One. Afterwards, compare it to the first or subsequent ones you have completed. Has your pain level changed? Did you notice that some tools worked better than others on aspects of your pain? It may be helpful to journal and look at what you have been able to change, as well as what you may have decided to live with *instead* of change. Have you used all of the tools? Have you used self-hypnosis or hypnosis to assist in this process? Let's look at what else may be helpful for you.

Reiki, Massage, and Other Body Work

In the field of integrative medicine, there are many helpful modalities and healing tools, and I am most familiar with Reiki. The knowledge that an unseen energy flows through all living things and is connected directly to the quality of health has been part of the wisdom of many cultures since ancient times and discussed at length in this writing. We have seen how the existence of this life force energy has been verified by recent scientific experiments, and medical doctors are considering the role it plays in the functioning of the immune system and the healing process.

Reiki is a form of laying on of hands healing. Its origins have been traced to Tibet. The word *Reiki* is made of two Japanese words–*Rei*, which refers to God's Wisdom or the Higher Power, and *Ki*, which is life force energy. So Reiki is actually life force energy. In China, this energy is called *chi* or *qi*; it is known as *prana* in India, *mana* in Hawaii, and *orenda* in Native American cultures. Another name for this energy is *aura*, which is the electrical force field that surrounds the physical body.

Reiki is used to apply life force energy to relieve pain, promote the healing process, revitalize, regenerate, and calm. It differs somewhat from touch healing in that the position of the hands over (or on) the body aligns more closely with the chakras.

Disease begins first on a non-physical level and then manifests on the physical level. Reiki will stimulate the aura and heal at that level. Lack of vitality is the cause of dis-ease in the non-physical, and Reiki stimulates the life force energy in the aura, giving the body more energy and vitality as well. Reiki eases trauma and shock, reduces stress and pain, and keeps tissue damage to a minimum. Your body holds the cellular memory of perfect health within. Reiki assists the body in remembering this perfect health. It is especially helpful for renewal when you find yourself too busy and working without rest. It is a technique for stress reduction and relaxation that allows everyone to tap into an unlimited supply of life force energy to improve health and enhance the quality of life.

An amazingly simple technique to learn, the ability to use Reiki is not taught in the usual sense, but is instead transferred to the student by the Reiki Master. Its use is not dependent on one's intellectual capacity or spiritual development and, therefore, is available to everyone. It has been successfully taught to thousands of people of all ages and backgrounds.

A Reiki treatment feels like a wonderful glowing radiance that flows through you and surrounds you. Reiki treats the whole person, including body, emotions, mind, and spirit. It creates many beneficial effects including relaxation and feelings of peace, security, and well-being. Many have reported miraculous results. Reiki is a simple, natural, and safe method of spiritual healing and self-improvement that everyone can use. Whether you are receiving or giving a Reiki treatment, you get the benefits of Reiki. Some of the results are relaxation, pain relief, accelerated healing, balancing of the chakras and clearing of the aura, slower respiration, and lowering of the blood pressure for those who need it.

Healing Touch

Healing Touch is another energy therapy you may be interested in receiving or learning. It helps to balance your physical, mental, emotional, and spiritual well-being. Like Reiki, Healing Touch works with your energy field to support your natural ability to heal. Founded in 1989 by Janet Mentgen, an RN, Healing Touch was used as a continuing education program for nurses.[1] Today it is used widely in hospitals and other medical settings. You may find many of the massage therapists in your area are also Healing Touch practitioners.

After a car accident in 2006 in which I was rear-ended, I went to a massage therapist friend for treatment. She used Healing Touch on me, and I could immediately feel the energy shift and release. I was impressed. It took the kinks out of my muscles quickly, and I felt like myself again.

Massage Therapy

Many massage therapists will use different techniques to augment their practice, such as hot rock massage and massage with therapeutic oils, but massage alone is very beneficial. It can be a great preventative measure in addition to helping with pain relief. We addressed chi deficiency earlier, and massage can be helpful for this lack of energy. Also, the joints become less elastic as you age, and massage can help keep your muscles, joints, and ligaments more supple.

When I hurt my shoulder in London schlepping my bags around in and out of the Tube, a massage therapist was extremely helpful in releasing the pain and tension in the muscle, as well as teaching me how to employ a pillow while sleeping so the arm could be elevated a little and not strained as I slept. Massage is also very nurturing. If you live alone or don't receive touch, massage is a blessing.

Electromagnetic Protection

According to the online dictionary found at Dictionary.com **(http://www.dictionary.com)**, electro pollution is defined as:

> Nonionizing electromagnetic radiation propagated through the atmosphere by broadcast towers, radar installations, and microwave appliances, and the magnetic fields surrounding electrical appliances and power lines, which is believed to have polluting effects on people and the environment; also called electromagnetic smog.

In Week Ten, we discussed your biofield. Although there is much controversy over what will or will not help protect us from electromagnetic pollution, much of what I have read concludes that there is indeed a problem. Earlier I shared the story of how wearing a pendant helped me to quickly recover my energy and health. My understanding is that the vibrations coming from cell phones, televisions, microwaves, and other items that are plugged into the electrical system are man-made waves, not natural to the environment and not natural to the environment of the human energy field or biofield. The BioPro (now Gia Wellness) pendant supports my body's own self-healing ability by changing the vibration of the electropollution into a wave against which my body can defend itself. There are many studies that support this claim, and I encourage you to decide for yourself. You can learn more at **http://candess.inspiredwellness411.com**, use your newfound skill of kinesiology, your intuition, or find a combination of the three that works for you. If you decide to use products to protect you from the electromagnetic pollution, there are even more sources that you can find on the Internet.

If you choose not to explore this option, but do believe that electromagnetic pollution is dangerous, here are some things you can do:

1. If you have an electric clock or radio next to your head when you sleep, either get a battery clock or move the clock as far from your sleeping space as you can.

2. Unplug anything that you are not using.

3. If you do not want to unplug items, it is helpful to get power strips so you can plug several items into one strip and turn them all off at once. This works well with computers and printers.

4. If you use a microwave, stand several feet away from the microwave when you are using it.

5. Use land phones when possible, and do not let children use your cell phone.

6. Use headphones rather than Bluetooth earpieces.

Activating Your Energy

We become activated energetically in many ways. What I mean by this is that our vibration becomes increased — activated to a higher level. Think again of the scale I talked about in Week Eleven from David Hawkins's Map of Consciousness. You can calibrate your own vibration using this technique. One way you can become activated at a higher level is by being in nature. The energy of plants, trees, and water can activate you. Another way is matching or being around those who are vibrating at a higher level. You can also become activated by what you read, as I mentioned in Week Ten. When I feel a little low, I often listen to a CD by a spiritual teacher or mentor.

In 2009 I attended the Hay House "I Can Do It" at Sea – Alaska Cruise. During the cruise, I took a workshop on submitting a book proposal. The class was taught by the top marketing director and the top editing director of Hay House. The ship was full of over 1,200 spiritually minded people including Louise Hay, Gregg Braden, Sylvia Brown, Wayne Dyer, Caroline Myss, and Brian Weiss. The energy was incredibly high, and I am sure healing took place naturally on multiple levels for many of the participants as we matched and increased energies.

The more you put yourself in places where the vibration is high, the more you can activate your own energy. Think back over the last few years. Where did you find you were activated? Where did you lose energy?

Manifesting

What you focus on increases. This is a large part of manifesting. Use the following simple steps to bring what you truly desire into your life:

1. Imagine the END result. Be clear and specific about what you want to manifest. Ask yourself if having this manifestation will bring you more love, happiness, joy, peace, wisdom, or abundance.

2. Clearly IDENTIFY what you want. Write down what you would like to manifest. The Universe does not process negatives, so if you say "I don't want to lose money," the Universe will process this as "I want to lose money." Focus on the positive. It would be better to say, "I receive an abundance of wealth from the Universe. I have a wealth of love, friends, employment opportunities, money, and resources." You can rephrase this in the way that fits for you.

3. ENVISION what it is that you are manifesting. Use all of your senses. See yourself with this manifestation, hear it happening, taste what you would taste, feel it, and experience all the sensations of this manifestation. You are in a natural trance right before you fall asleep and when you first wake up. Imagine this manifestation at these times to increase the manifestation. Imagine what it feels like *right now* to have this manifestation!

4. Be RECEPTIVE. Maintain your desires, but be unattached to the specifics of the outcome. Once you give this to the Universe, understand that you may not understand how the Universe is creating this manifestation. Allow the Universe to work through people, situations, and institutions. Do not limit the Universe by being disappointed if the manifestation does not come on your timeline or in the way you expected. Because of free will, many people are involved in your manifestation!

5. Practice an ATTITUDE OF GRATITUDE! Be appreciative of what you have, and see every person and every situation as a possible solution to your manifestation. Be happy! See every day as an opportunity to grow and be grateful! Be generous with others.

6. RELEASE any fears or doubts regarding your deserving this manifestation. Let go of anything in the past that is holding you back. Forgive yourself and others for the past. Take

responsibility for your life today! Follow your heart and you will create what you desire.

7. RECEIVE what comes your way. Be aware of what is coming and be careful not to block the gifts of the Universe. Allow yourself to receive. The world is abundant. Claim your abundance and be generous.

Overall Health

You have been given a lot of information in this book, and I hope that you are able to reread sections and practice the tools and exercises so that they become daily habits in your life. In summary, ultimately, you create your health by your choices. The external world, including your body, acts as a mirror reflecting your inner beliefs and expectations. Your doing, thinking, and feeling affect all aspects of your physiology, which results in good health or disease, as well as happiness or depression.

The simplest and most productive way to feel good naturally is to meditate in the morning and early evening. Morning is also a good time to stretch, play, move your body, and check in with your body. Experience the outdoors as often as possible, and become conscious of your surroundings. Eat healthy food that is not processed, and eat the largest meal in the middle of the day. Avoid alcohol and other drugs, including sugar. Drink eight glasses of un-chlorinated water daily.

Experience and express your feelings. Take time to understand what you are feeling and the origin of the feeling. See a counselor or a body worker to help you release your feelings. Relax before bed with a book, bath, or some light organizing. Be positive in your thoughts, and allow yourself to belong, to be loving and forgiving, and to experience yourself in a process of health and healing. Take responsibility for your own health. And, I would like to add, be grateful!

Tools and Exercises

1. Ground yourself, close your eyes, and breathe deeply. Take a moment to imagine you have 100 circuits of energy emanating from the top of your head. See where your energy is going. You can do this by seeing what memories and feelings surface. Do a timed writing for twenty minutes to get more information.

2. Assess your home for electropollution. Research on the Internet what is said to be harmful, and take some precautions by investing in protective products or using the ideas I gave you in this week.

3. Make an appointment for Reiki, Healing Touch, massage, or another nurturing experience. If you do this kind of work as well, do not trade sessions. Allow yourself to receive.

4. Go to your local independent bookstore and spend some time looking through the books. Allow your intuition to take you to the book that will be activating for you.

The whole process of self-healing involves becoming conscious and activating your own life force energy and directing it consciously. Have fun with this. Use the tools that you find to be the most helpful and share them with friends. If you need more support, find my coaching program on my website http://www.CandessCampbell.com or contact a mental health therapist to guide you through this information. You may even want to get a group together to go through the book and share with each other.

There are a couple of points I have not yet made, but I find them to be very important. The first is to be sure to forgive yourself for anything you may be holding without letting go. Forgive others as well, because as we hold resentments of the past, the resentments hold us much tighter. The second is a word I have learned to love as I embrace it. The word is *surrender*. The more I have learned to surrender my will to God, the Universe, the Divine ... the simpler my life has become. When you understand that you are not alone, that there is a part of you that is much wiser and much more capable, it becomes easier to let go and trust that your own Higher Self, your Inner Guide, the Holy Spirit will create for you in a manner beyond what you could imagine yourself.

"Doctor, I'd like a bottle of placebo please."

– Candess M. Campbell

Appendix 1: Relaxation Induction Script

(*Note*: This is a general script. Please change it to fit your needs.)

Take a moment to get into a comfortable position ... let yourself relax and feel yourself supported by the chair ... let's take a deep breath together ... now take another deep breath and feel your abdomen expand as you gently exhale. Allow your eyes to become heavy and close.

For the next few minutes I'd like you to listen to the sound of my voice ... and as you listen ... you may want to let your body begin to slow itself down ... nice and easy ... let all the stress and the strain of the day fade away.

You are beginning to relax ... to let go ... and slow down. Let go of your body tension ... feeling relaxed ... let go of your body tension right now ... as you listen with your mind.

A flow of relaxation makes it way down from the top of your head ... all the way down to the tips of your toes. You begin to relax ... to feel your muscles letting go ... they seem to just melt.

Your breathing is natural and effortless ... you are beginning to slow down and to relax. Let all the negative feelings fade away ... let the world fade away.

It feels good having relaxation move through your body ... a wave of relaxation ... and it begins at the very top of your head. You allow your scalp to relax ... and the relaxation flows downward across your forehead ... through your eyebrows and eyes ... down to your cheeks and nose ... and across your mouth. You even let your jaw relax a little bit as you unclench your teeth.

You are practicing letting go of your body tension ... it helps you to open your mind to your inner feelings and your inner thoughts. As you listen even more ... let the relaxation flow ... just imagine more and more relaxation flowing gently downward from your face into your neck ... and let go ... and relax.

It's a slowing down that flows deep within you ... just imagine this flow of relaxation spreading out across your shoulders ... and down through your arms. Relaxation flows through your upper arms ... through your lower arms ... and moves down into your hands, your fingers, and your fingertips.

Imagine all the tight, tense feelings from your upper body are melting right out the tips of your fingers ... your upper body is letting go as you let the relaxation flow deeper and downward. All tensions and all negative feelings fade away ... and you relax even more through your chest and upper back ... and now down your stomach.

You may even imagine that each time you take a breath in, you breathe in even more relaxation. And each time you breathe out, you let go of all tension. Just let all the negative feelings fade away ... as you continue to unwind and relax.

Imagine this wave of relaxation moving gently down into your lower back ... now down into your hips ... your thighs ... which just seem to melt ... and you let it happen ... you feel the tension leaving your body. You feel heavy and relaxed.

Your eyes are closed, but your inner mind is open ... you are listening to all the suggestions, all the thoughts, and all the ideas that are going to help you reach your goal.

Appendix 2: NLP Word List

Visual

Bright	Dull	Illuminate	Picture
Brilliant	Fuzzy	Imagine	Shiny
Clear	Glimpse	Look	View
Colorful	Hazy		Vivid

Auditory

Amplify	Harmony	Melody	Roar
Bang	Hear	Noisy	Scream
Call	Listen	Pitch	Tone
Discuss	Loud	Quiet	

Kinesthetic

Abrasive	Pain	Relaxed	Tense
Clammy	Penetrating	Rough	Tingle
Firm	Pressure	Smooth	Vibrations
Moist	Tender	Soft	

Olfactory

Acrid	Fishy	Pine	Smoky
Aroma	Floral	Rancid	Stink
Burnt	Fragrant	Reek	Vapor
Citrus	Minty	Smell	

Gustatory

Acidic	Carbonated	Pungent	Stale
Bitter	Fresh	Salty	Sweet
Bland	Fruity	Sour	Taste
Buttery	Nutty	Spicy	

Appendix 3: Building a Vocabulary for Feelings

Often we use words which describe how we interpret others' behavior, rather than the emotions we are experiencing. (Example: abandoned, abused, attacked, betrayed, boxed-in, bullied, cheated, coerced, co-opted, cornered, diminished, distrusted, interrupted, intimidated, and let down are not feelings, but interpretations of another's behavior).

Here is a list of words which describe how we are likely to feel when our needs are being met:

Adventurous	Contented	Glad
Affectionate	Cool	Glorious
Alert	Curious	Good-humored
Alive	Delighted	Grateful
Amazed	Eager	Happy
Appreciative	Ecstatic	Helpful
Aroused	Encouraged	Hopeful
Astonished	Energetic	Inquisitive
Blissful	Engrossed	Inspired
Calm	Enlivened	Intense
Carefree	Enthusiastic	Interested
Cheerful	Excited	Involved
Comfortable	Expansive	Joyous, joyful
Complacent	Fascinated	Keyed-up
Composed	Free	Loving
Concerned	Friendly	Mellow
Confident	Fulfilled	Moved

Optimistic	Refreshed	Thankful
Overjoyed	Relaxed	Thrilled
Overwhelmed	Relieved	Touched
Peaceful	Satisfied	Tranquil
Pleasant	Sensitive	Trusting
Pleased	Serene	Upbeat
Proud	Stimulated	Warm
Quiet	Surprised	Wonderful
Radiant	Tender	Zestful

Here is a list of words to describe how we are likely to feel when our needs are not being met:

Aggravated	Cool	Exhausted
Agitated	Cross	Fearful
Angry	Dejected	Fidgety
Annoyed	Depressed	Frightened
Anxious	Detached	Frustrated
Apathetic	Disenchanted	Furious
Apprehensive	Disappointed	Gloomy
Ashamed	Discouraged	Guilty
Beat	Disgusted	Harried
Bitter	Disheartened	Helpless
Blue	Distressed	Hesitant
Bored	Disturbed	Horrified
Brokenhearted	Downhearted	Horrible
Cold	Dull	Hostile
Concerned	Edgy	Hot
Confused	Embarrassed	Hurt

Impatient	Nervous	Shocked
Indifferent	Numb	Skeptical
Intense	Overwhelmed	Startled
Irritated	Panicky	Surprised
Jealous	Passive	Suspicious
Keyed-up	Pessimistic	Terrified
Lazy	Puzzled	Troubled
Listless	Reluctant	Uncomfortable
Lonely	Repelled	Unhappy
Mad	Resentful	Upset
Mean	Restless	Weary
Miserable	Sad	Withdrawn
Mournful	Scared	Worried
	Sensitive	Wretched

Words like *ignored* express how we *interpret others*, rather than how we feel. Here is a sampling of such words:

Abandoned	Co-opted	Misunderstood
Abused	Cornered	Neglected
Attacked	Diminished	Overworked
Betrayed	Distrusted	Patronized
Boxed-in	Interrupted	Pressured
Bullied	Intimidated	Provoked
Cheated	Let down	Put down
Coerced	Manipulated	Rejected

Taken for	Unappreciated	Unsupported
granted	Unheard	Unwanted
Threatened	Unseen	Used

Note: Source: Nonviolent Communication: A Language of Life
© by Dr. Marshall Rosenberg, 2003 - published by PuddleDancer Press.
for more information visit www.CNVC.org and
www.NonviolentCommunication.com

Appendix 4: Symptoms of Trauma

The nervous system compensates for being in a state of self-perpetuating arousal by setting off a chain of adaptations that eventually bind and organize the energy into "symptoms."(146) These adaptations function as a safety valve to the nervous system. The first symptoms of trauma usually appear shortly after the event that engendered them. Others will develop over time.

The first symptoms to appear:

- *Hyperarousal to prepare for a potential threat which may include increased heartbeat, increased breathing, agitation, difficulty sleeping, tension, muscular jitteriness, racing thoughts and anxiety attacks. (pp. 132-133)*

- *Constriction to assure focus toward the threat such as altered breathing, muscle tone and posture. The blood vessels constrict so more blood can go to the tensed muscles for defensive action. (p. 135)*

- *Dissociation (including denial)*

- *Feelings of helplessness*

Other early symptoms that begin to show up at the same time or shortly after those above are:

- *Hypervigilance (being "on guard" at all times)*
- *Intrusive images or flashbacks*
- *Extreme sensitivity to light and sound*

- *Hyperactivity*
- *Exaggerated emotional and startle responses*
- *Nightmares and night terrors*
- *Abrupt mood swings: e.g., rage reactions or temper tantrums, shame*
- *Reduced ability to deal with stress (easily and frequently stressed out)*
- *Difficulty sleeping*

Note: From *Waking the Tiger: Healing Trauma* by Peter A. Levine, published by North Atlantic Books, copyright © 1997 by Peter A. Levine. Reprinted by permission of publisher.

Appendix 5: Trauma Questionnaire

Have you ever had something traumatic happen to you or to someone close to you? This could be something that happened one time, but had a severe effect, or something that happened more than once over a period of time. The events could be things like sexual, physical, or emotional abuse; serious illness or injury; unexpected sudden loss or several losses; or violent acts toward you or witnessed by you toward someone you care about.

Please answer the following questions using this scale:

0 = Not at all
1 = Once a week or less, a little bit, or once in a while
2 = 2 to 4 times a week, somewhat, half the time
3 = 5 or more times a week, very much, almost always

1. Do you have thoughts about what happened when you don't want these thoughts? _____

2. Do you have bad dreams or nightmares about what happened? _____

3. Do you feel like it is happening again when something reminds you of the experience? _____

4. Do you get emotionally upset when you are reminded of what happened? (see question 17)

_____

5. Have you been trying not to feel or think about what happened? _____
   What do you do to stop it? (Write your response in your journal.)

6. Have you stayed away from places or stopped doing things that remind you of what happened? _____ What do you do or not do? (Write your response in your journal.)

7. Are there parts of what happened that you can't remember but think were important? _____

8. Have you stopped doing things that you liked doing before the experience? _____

9. Did the traumatic experience change the way you think your future will turn out now? _____

10. Do you feel alone or lonely since the experience? _____

11. Do you feel numb or as if you don't have feelings? _____

12. Have you had a lot of trouble falling asleep or staying asleep? _____

13. Have you been more irritable, crankier, or have you been mad a lot more since the trauma? _____

14. Have you been having trouble concentrating? _____

15. Are you worried that something bad is going to happen to you? _____

16. Have you been jumpier, more easily startled, or more on guard since it happened? _____

17. Have you had physical reactions when reminded of what happened (sweating, fast heartbeat, nervous feeling, etc.)? _____

Please take time to journal about memories or thoughts that surface as you answer the questions. If your answers are related to a trauma and your score is 10 or more, I strongly suggest you find a mental health therapist to help you heal the origin of the trauma.

I especially recommend therapists who are trained in hypnotherapy and have experience with trauma clients, or therapists who are trained in EMDR. You can find these in appendix 9: Trauma and Healing Resources.

Note: Created by Candess M. Campbell, PhD.

Appendix 6: The Bagua Map for Feng Shui

Wealth and Prosperity	Fame	Love and Marriage
Abundance Manifesting Receiving	Your Reputation What You Are Famous For	Marriage Partnerships Feminine
Wood	Fire	Earth
Blues, Purples & Reds	Reds	Reds, Pinks & White
Family	Health	Creativity and Children
New Beginnings Initiations Health	Balance Unity Centeredness	Creative Expression Conception Ability to Complete
Wood	Earth	Metal
Blues & Greens	Yellow & Earth Tones	Whites & Pastels
Knowledge and Self-Cultivation	Career	Helpful People and Travel
Understanding Spirituality Self-Awareness	Life Path Communication Social Connections Wisdom	Benefactors Support Network Masculine
Earth	Water	Metal
Black, Blues & Greens	Black & Dark Tones	Whites, Grays & Black

Note: Feng Shui Map created by Candess M. Campbell, PhD

You can also find this Bagua Map at
http://candesscampbell.com/books/self-help-tools/feng-shui-bagua-map

Appendix 7: Chakra Stems

First Chakra Sentence Stems

- My parents still believe ...
- What I thought was important when I was 10 years old was ...
- What I want to teach my children is ...
- The strangest superstition I have is ...
- What I value most is ...
- I would never ...
- I compromised myself when I ...
- What still hurts from childhood is ...
- I was so embarrassed when ...
- My relationship with my mother is ...
- My relationship with my father is ...
- What is unfinished from childhood is ...
- Traditions that are important to me are ...
- I need others most when ...
- The tribe I belong to most is ...
- What I am afraid to say is ...
- What I am afraid to write is ...
- What comforts me the most is ...

Second Chakra Sentence Stems

- The most powerful choice I have made is ...
- The scariest choice I have made is ...

- The relationship that empowers me most is with …
- The relationship where I lose the most power is …
- I compromise myself when I need …
- A sexual woman is …
- A sexual man is …
- My sexuality feels …
- When I have money, I feel …
- When I have no money, I feel …
- When I spend large amounts of money spontaneously, I feel …
- Rich people are …
- Poverty is a sign of …
- If I had a million dollars to spend immediately, I would …
- I feel most powerful when …
- It is totally unethical to …
- I feel seductive when …
- The person I control most is …
- The person who controls me most is …
- I need to call my spirit back from …

Third Chakra Sentence Stems

- What I like about myself is …
- What I don't like about myself is …
- What I want to change about myself is …
- I'll never change my …
- I'm honest when it comes to …

- I am dishonest about ...
- I'm critical when it comes to ...
- I protect myself by...
- The person I blame the most is ...
- The person who gives me feedback about myself is ...
- I accept feedback from ...
- I learn from feedback from ...
- What others don't understand about me is ...
- Others are critical of me about ...
- I need approval from ...
- The person I didn't like but spent time with was ...
- I know I should ...
- I can't seem to continue to ...
- I know I shouldn't ...
- I am afraid of ...
- I feel responsible for ...
- I feel responsible to ...
- I wish my life were more ...
- I wish my life were less ...
- The person who wants my approval the most is ...
- I am weakest when ...
- I am strongest when ...
- I don't take care of myself when I ...
- I take care of myself by ...
- I don't stick to my commitments when ...

- I feel responsible for others when …
- I avoid responsibility by …
- What I can change in my life is …
- What I will change today is …

Now identify what you want …

- What do I want?
- What am I doing now?
- Is it working?
- What is my plan? (specific and measurable with dated outcomes)

Note: Created by Candess M. Campbell, PhD

You can find more sentence stems in my upcoming book *Sentence Stems: Empowerment by Turning Yourself Inside Out!*

Appendix 8: Kinesiology Testing Steps

1. **Circuit Fingers**

   Use your non-dominant hand and place your hand palm up. Connect the tip of your middle finger with your thumb. When doing this 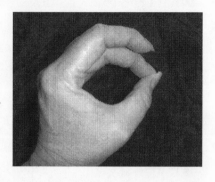 you have closed an electrical circuit in your hand, and it is this circuit you will use for testing.

2. **Test Fingers**

   Now take the middle finger of your dominant hand and place it in the circle you have formed, with the top joint of your dominant 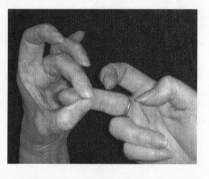 hand touching where your middle finger and thumb of your non-dominant hand meet. You will be gently pulling this middle finger toward you when we test, either breaking the connection between the middle finger and the thumb, or not.

3. **Positive and Negative Response**

Now, keeping your hands in this testing position, make a statement where you know the answer is yes. You may say, 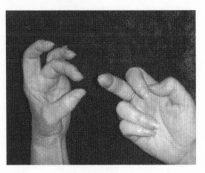 "My name is _____." After making the statement, pull toward yourself with your middle finger of the dominant hand and see what happens. If it is a true statement, the middle finger and thumb will remain strong. Now, make a statement that is false, such as, "My name is Mickey Mouse." Again, pull toward yourself with your middle finger of the dominant hand with the same amount of force. With this false statement, the circuit of the middle finger and the thumb will break.

Play with this testing for a while. At first you may feel awkward, like you are making it happen, but over time you will get the sense of how to do this. Be sure to make declarative statements, rather than asking questions.

Once you feel secure about the process, you can go on to ask questions you do not know the answers to. Be sure to use the same amount of force for both hands and be gentle about it, not forcing too hard, but sensing the break in the circuit.

If you have difficulty with this process, you may be dehydrated. Drink a large glass of water. Also, you may need to get your energy crossing correctly, so practice the Cross Crawl technique by Donna Eden, which I explained in Week Eleven in the Kinesiology and Muscle testing section.

Note: From Candess M. Campbell, Ph.D. © Kinesiology Self Test *08-03-2009*

Appendix 9: Trauma and Healing Resources

Candess's websites for further information on *12 Weeks to Self-Healing: Transforming Pain through Energy Medicine*:
http://www.12Weeksto SelfHealing.com
http://on.fb.me/Candess
http://www.CandessCampbell.com

The Empowerment Group, LLC
75-6099 Kuakini Highway
Kailua-Kona, HI 96740
Toll free: 800.800.MIND (6463)
http://www.hypnosis.com

EMDR Institute, Inc.
PO Box 750
Watsonville, CA 95077
USA Tel: 831-761-1040
Fax: 831-761-1204
http://www.emdr.com

Institute of Spiritual Healing and Aromatherapy
P.O. Box 741239
Arvada, Colorado 80006
303-467-7829

Young Living Essential Oils
Thanksgiving Point Business Park
3125 Executive Parkway
Lehi, Utah 84043
http://cc.younglivingworld.com

Mountain Rose Herbs
PO Box 50220
Eugene, OR 97405
http://www.mountainroseherbs.com

Alcoholics Anonymous
http://www.aa.org/

Narcotics Anonymous
http://www.na.org/

Al-Anon
http://www.al-anon.alateen.org/

Overeaters Anonymous
http://www.oa.org/

Gamblers Anonymous
http://www.gamblersanonymous.org/ga/index.php

ENDNOTES

Preface

1. Cameron, J. 1992. *The Artist's Way: A Spiritual Path to Higher Creativity*. New York: Penguin Putnam Publishing.

How to Use This Book

1. Moss, M.S.W., Ph.D, P.C.C., L. E. 2011. Professional Certified Coach and Course Creator, Institute For Life Coach Training.

2. Mauer, Ph.D. R. 2004. *One Small Step Can Change your Life: The Kaizen Way*. New York: Workman Publishing Company.

3. Goldburg, N. 1986. *Writing Down the Bones*. Boston: Shambhala.

4. Smyth, J.; Stone, A.; Hurewitz, A.; & Kaell, A.(1999). "Effects of writing about stressful experiences on symptom reduction in patients with asthma or rheumatoid arthritis: A randomized trial." *Journal of the American Medical Association*, 281(14): 1304-1309.

Week One: Evaluate Your Situation

1. Glasser, W. 1998. Realty Therapy certification workshop by The William Glasser Institute. **http://www.wglasser.com.**

2. Boffey, Ed.D. D.B. 1997. *Reinventing Yourself,* 3rd printing 1997. Available from New View Publications, Chapel Hill, NC **info@newviewpublications.com** 1-800-441-3604.

3. Ibid.

4. Amen, D. G. 2008. *Magnificent Mind at Any Age: Natural Ways to Unleash Your Brain's Maximum Potential.* New York: Crown Publishing Group.

5. Ibid.

6. Amen, D.G. Amen Brain System Test. **http://www.amenclinics.com.**

7. Walsh, Ph.D. B. n.d. *Sensory Description of Pain.* [Unpublished handout].

8. Radha, S.S. 2004. *Realities of the Dreaming Mind: The Practice of Dream Yoga,* 2nd ed. Spokane, WA: Timeless Books.

9. Taylor, J. 1993. *Where People Fly and Water Runs Uphill: Using Dreams to Tap the Wisdom of the Unconscious.* New York: Warner Books, Inc.

10. Myss, C. & Shealy, N. 2005. Medical Intuition Training workshop. Virginia Beach, VA. October.

11. Virtue, D. 2008. Angel Therapy Practitioner® Course. Kailua-Kona, Hawaii. Angel Therapy Inc. **http://angeltherapy.com.**

Week Two: Finding Your Passion

1. Bolker, J. Ed.D. 1998. *Writing Your Dissertation in Fifteen Minutes a Day: A Guide to Starting, Revising, and Finishing Your Doctoral Thesis.* New York: Holt Paperbacks.

2. Beattie, M. 1992. *Codependent No More.* Center City, MN: Hazelton Foundation.

3. Gray, J. 2004. *Men Are from Mars, Women Are from Venus: The Classic Guide to Understanding the Opposite Sex.* New York: Harper Collins.

4. Chapman, Ph.D. G. 2010. *The Five Love Languages.* Chicago: Northfield Publishing.

Week Three: Rule Out and Make Changes

1. Dick-Kronenberg, N.D., L. The Windrose Naturopathic Clinic. 1137 W. Garland Ave Spokane WA 99205. 509 327-5143. **http://www.windroseclinic.com.**

2. Ibid.

3. Dick-Kronenberg, N.D., L. Song of Health Food Intolerance Information. **http://www.windroseclinic.com/links.html**.

4. Gia Wellness. **http://www.giawellness.com/candess. http://candess.inspiredwellness411.com/**.

5. Mendel, C. Moffat, Colorado.

6. Dyro, F. M. 2006. "Organophosphates." *eMedicine*. **http://emedicine.medscape .com/article/1175139-overview**.

7. O'Brien, M. 1990. "Are pesticides taking away the ability of our children to learn?" *Journal of Pesticide Reform*. Vol. 10, No. 4, Winter 1990 – 1991: 4-8. **http://eap.mcgill.ca/MagRack/JPR/JPR_08.htm**.

8. Heritage, J. 2004. "The Fate of Transgenes in the Human Gut." *Nature BioTechnology*. Vol. 22 (2): 170-172.

9. Netherwood, T.; Martin-Orue, S. M.; O'Donnell, A. G.; Gockling, S.; Graham, J.; Mathers, J. C. & Gilbert, H. J. 2004. "Assessing the survival of transgenic plant DNA in the human gastrointestinal tract." *Nature Biotechnology*, Vol. 22(2):204-209.

10. Watrud, L. S.; Lee, E. H.; Fairbrother, A.; Burdick, C.; Reichman, J. R.; Bollman, M.; Storm, M.; King, G. & Van dewater, P. K. 2004. "Evidence for Landscape-Level, Pollen-Mediated Gene Flow from Genetically Modified Creeping Bentgrass with CP4 EPSPS as a Marker." *National Academy of Sciences*, 101(40): 14533-14538.

11. United States Department of Agriculture. 2008. "Organic Labeling and Marketing Information." *United States Department of Agriculture Agricultural Marketing Service*. **http://www.ams.usda.gov/amsv1.0/getfile?dDocName=stel dev3004446&acct=nopgeninfo**.

12. Virtue, D. & Prelitz, B. 2001. *Eating In The Light: Making the Switch to Vegetarianism on Your Spiritual Path*. Carlsbad, CA: Hay House. 27-29.

13. Ibid.

14. Ibid.

15. Solochek, D. & Zeff, N.D., J. "The O.G. Carroll Food Intolerance Test from the Carroll Method." *National College of Natural Medicine.*

16. Maliniak, P., e-mail communication to author, May 22, 2012.

17. Scarito, P., e-mail communication to author, May 22, 2012.

18. Radha Yoga Center/ADHP. 406 S. Coeur d'Alene St., Suite C, Spokane, WA 99201. **http://www.radhayoga.org/**.

Week Four: Hypnotherapy

1. Alman, B. M. & Lambrou, P. 1983. *Self-Hypnosis: The Complete Manual for Health and Self-Change.* 2nd ed. Philadelphia: Brunner/Mazel Publishers. 8-9.

2. Ibid.

3. Ibid.

4. Simonton, O. C.; Matthews-Simonton, S. & Creighton, JL. 1992. *Getting Well Again.* New York: Bantam Books. 187.

5. Kostere, K. & Malatesta, L. 1989. *Get The Results You Want: A Guide to Communication Excellence for the Helping Professional.* Lake Oswego, OR: Metamorphous Press.

6. Sele, H. 1952. *The Story of the Adaptation Syndrome.* Montreal, Quebec, Canada: Acta Inc.

7. Alman, B. M. & Lambrou, P. 1983. *Self-Hypnosis: The Complete Manual for Health and Self-Change* (2nd ed.). Philadelphia: Brunner/Mazel Publishers. 166.

8. Simonton et al., *Getting Well Again*.

9. Ibid., 148.

10. Alman & Lambrou. *Self-Hypnosis*.

11. Kazlev, M. A. 1999. "Jung's Conception of the Collective Unconscious." **http://www.kheper.net/topics/Jung/collective_unconscious .html.**

12. Simonton et al., *Getting Well Again*, 148.

13. Ibid., 141.

14. Ibid., 31.

15. Ibid., 148.

16. Glasser, W. 1998. *Choice Theory: A New Psychology for Personal Freedom*. New York: HarperCollins.

Week Five: Assess Your Beliefs

1. Earth Stewards. **http://www.earthstewards.org/**.

2. Cameron, J. 1992. *The Artist's Way: A Spiritual Path to Higher Creativity*. New York: Penguin Putnam Publishing.

3. Lipton, B. 2005. *The Biology of Belief: Unleashing the Power of Consciousness, Matter and Miracles*. Santa Rosa, CA: Elite Books. 50-51.

4. Ibid.

5. Ibid.

6. The Fairy Congress. **http://www. fairycongress.com**.

7. Virtue, D. 2007. *How to Hear Your Angels*. Carlsbad, CA: Hay House, Inc.

8. Ibid., 47-48.

9. Ibid., 88.

10. Ibid., 115.

11. Ibid.

12. Ibid.

13. Ibid.

14. Ibid.

15. Ibid., 103-105.

16. Mesich, K. 2000. *The Sensitive Person's Survival Guide: An Alternative Health Answer to Emotional Sensitivity & Depression*. Lincoln, NE: iUniverse.

17. Ibid., 2.

18. Ibid., 3.

19. Ibid., 4.

20. Ibid.

21. Ibid., 5.

22. Ibid.

23. Ibid., 7.

24. Ibid., 8.

25. Ibid., 10.

26. Ibid., 10.

27. Ibid., 20.

28. Ibid., 20.

29. Glasser, *Choice Theory*.

30. Myss, C. & Shealy, N. 2005. Medical Intuition Training workshop. Virginia Beach, VA.

31. Chopra, D. 1990. *Quantum Healing: Exploring the Frontiers of Mind/Body Medicine*. New York: Bantam Books. 135.

32. Ibid., 140.

33. Ibid., 144.

34. Ibid., 150.

35. Ibid., 151.

36. Ibid., 169.

37. Ibid., 178.

38. Ibid.

39. Ibid.

40. Ibid., 179.

41. Ibid.

42. Lipton, B. 2005. *The Biology of Belief: Unleashing the Power of Consciousness, Matter and Miracles*. Santa Rosa, CA: Elite Books. 164.

43. Ibid., 165.

44. Ibid.

45. Ibid., 166.

46. Gerber, R. 2001. *Vibrational Medicine: The #1 Handbook of Subtle-Energy Therapies*. Rochester, VT: Bear & Company. 322, 351, 528-530.

47. Ibid.

48. Ibid., 530.

49. NVisable. 2012. **http://www.nvisible.com**.

50. Campbell, C.Ph.D. 1990. Chakra clearing. [Compact Disc]. **http://www.energymedicinedna.com**.

51. Gerber, *Vibrational Medicine*, 322.

Week Six: Stress Comes in Many Forms

1. Holmes, T.H.; Rahe, R.H. 1967. "The Social Readjustment Rating Scale." J Psychosom Res 11 (2): 213–8. **http://en.wikipedia.org/wiki/Holmes_and_Rahe _stress_scale**.

2. Rahe, R.H.; Mahan, J.L.; Arthur, R.J. 1970. "Prediction of Near-Future Health Change from Subjects' Preceding Life Changes." *Journal of Psychosomatic Research*. Vol.14. Issue 4: 401–6.

Week Seven: Feel Your Feelings

1. Hay, L. 2009. *Heal Your Body: The Mental Causes of Physical Disease and the Metaphysical Way to Overcome Them.* Rev. ed., 3rd ed. Carlsbad, CA: Hay House. 2.

2. Byrne, R. 2007. *The Secret* movie. **http://thesecret.tv/**.

3. Gerber, *Vibrational Medicine*, 351.

4. Truman, K. K. 2000. *Feelings Buried Alive Never Die*. St. George, UT: Olympus Distributing. 8.

5. Ibid., 10-11.

6. Ibid.

7. Lipton, *The Biology of Belief*, 164.

8. Ibid., 162.

9. Ibid., 163.

10. Ibid., 164.

11. Ibid., 165.

12. Ibid.

13. Ibid., 168-170.

14. Ibid., 165-166.

15. Myss, C. 1996. *Anatomy of the Spirit.* New York: Three Rivers Press. 103.

16. EMDR Institute Inc. 2011. "What is EMDR?" **http://www.emdr.com/ general-information/what-is-emdr.html**.

17. Flora, M.E. 2002. *Healing: Key to Spiritual Balance.* Everett, WA: CDM Publications. 47-51.

18. Ruby, M. 2000. "DNA Reprocessing and Reprogramming" class. *Possibilities Vocational School.* **http://www.possibilitiesdna.com/margaret.html**.

19. Beattie, M. 1986. *Codependent No More - How to Stop Controlling Others and Start Caring for Yourself.* 2nd ed. Center City, MN: Hazelden Publishing.

20. Essential Peacemaking: Women and Men ©Facilitators Manual. Earthstewarts Network, P.O. Box 10697, Bainbridge Island, WA 98110.

21. Ibid., 18.

22. Ibid., 34.

23. Rosenberg, M.B. 2003. *Nonviolent Communication: A Language of Life.* 2nd ed. Encinitas, CA: PuddleDancer Press. 44-45. **http://www.NonviolentCommunication.com**.

24. Ibid., 7

25. Flora, M.E. 2000. *Meditation: Key to Spiritual Awakening.* 2nd ed. Everett, WA: CDM Publications.

26. Rosenberg, *Nonviolent Communication.*

Week Eight: Prayer and Meditation

1. International Association of Spiritual Healers and Earth Stewards.

2. Dossey, L. 1993. *Healing Words: The Power of Prayer and the Practice of Medicine.* New York: HarperCollins.

3. Ibid., 91.

4. Flora, *Healing: Key to Spiritual Balance,* 13

5. Chopra, D. 1990. *Quantum Healing: Exploring the Frontiers of Mind/Body Medicine.* New York: Bantam Books. 178-179.

6. Ibid.

7. Rhada, S.S. 2004. *Kundalini: Yoga for the West.* Kootenay Bay, BC Canada: Timeless Books. 210- 211.

8. Church of Divine Man. 2402 Summit Ave. Everett, WA. 98201. 425-258-1449. 800-360-6509.

9. Rajhans, G. n.d. "The Power of Mantra Chanting: Why and How to Chant." **http://hinduism.about.com/od/prayersmantras/a/mantrachanting.htm**.

10. Ibid., Para 4.

11. Wikipedia. *Mantra.* **http://en.wikipedia.org/wiki/Mantra**.

12. Kabat-Zinn, J. 1994. *Wherever You Go, There You Are: Mindfulness Meditation in Everyday Life.* New York: Hyperion.

13. McCraken, L. M.; Gauntlett-Gilbert, J. & Vowles, K. 2006. "The Role of Mindfulness in a Contextual Cognitive-Behavioral Analysis of Chronic Pain-Related Suffering and Disability." *National Center for Biotechnology Information.*

http://www.ncbi
.nlm.nih.gov/pubmed/17257755?dopt=AbstractPlus.

14. Campbell, Ph.D. C. *Chakra Clearing CD.*
http://candesscampbell.com/products /chakra-clearing-cd.

Week Nine: Healing and Trauma

1. Levine, P. A., & Frederick, A. 1997. *Waking the Tiger: Healing Trauma: The Innate Capacity to Transform Overwhelming Experiences.* Berkeley, CA: North Atlantic Books.

2. Ibid., 51.

3. American Psychiatric Association. 2000. *Desk Reference to the Diagnostic Criteria From DSM-IV-TR.* Arlington, VA: American Psychiatric Publishing, Inc. 218-219.

4. Shapiro, F. 2006. "Eye Movement and Desensitization Reprocessing Training Manual Part 1." Rev. ed. Watsonville, CA: EMDR Institute, Inc.

5. Wikipedia. *Hypervigilance.*
http://en.wikipedia.org/wiki/Hypervigilance. para.1.

6. Shapiro, *Eye Movement and Desensitization Reprocessing Training Manual.*

7. Ibid., 14.

8. Ibid.

9. Shapiro, F. & Forrest, M. S. 1997,2004. *EMDR The Breakthrough "Eye Movement" Therapy for Overcoming Anxiety, Stress and Trauma.* Cambridge, MA: Basic Books. 14

10. Shapiro, *Eye Movement and Desensitization Reprocessing Training Manual,* 14-15.

11. Levine & Frederick, *Waking the Tiger*, 161.

12. Bass, E. & Davis, L. 2004. *The Courage to Heal: A Guide for Women Survivors of Childhood Sexual Abuse.* New York: HarperCollins. 39-43.

13. Levine & Frederick, *Waking the Tiger*, 165.

14. Ibid., 164.

15. Ibid.

16. Shapiro, F. 2001. *Eye Movement Desensitization Reprocessing: Basic Principles, Protocols, and Procedures.* 2nd ed. New York: The Guilford Press. xiii-xiv.

17. Ibid., 9-10.

18. Ibid.

19. Ibid., 74.

20. Shapiro, *Eye Movement and Desensitization Reprocessing Training Manual,* 80

21. The William Glasser Institute. **http://www.wglasser.com/**.

22. The EMDR International Association. **http://www.emdria.org/**.

23. Shapiro, *Eye Movement Desensitization Reprocessing: Basic Principles,* 32.

24. Touch for Health. **http://www.touch4health.com/**.

Week Ten: Your Energy System

1. Collinge, W. 1998. *Subtle Energy: Awakening to the Unseen Forces in Our Lives.* New York: Warner Books.

2. Ibid., 2.

3. Collinge, *Subtle Energy*.

4. Institute of HeartMath. **http://www.heartmath.org/**.

5. Collinge, *Subtle Energy*, 4-5.

6. Ibid.

7. Ibid.

8. Ibid., 11.

9. Ibid.

10. Ibid., 7.

11. Ibid.

12. Ibid.

13. Ibid., 12.

14. Ibid.

15. Ibid.,13.

16. Tchi, Rodika. n.d. "What is Feng Shui – Feng Shui theory and Feng Shui tools." **http://fengshui.about.com/od/thebasics/qt/fengshui.htm**. Para 3-4.

17. Ibid.

18. Collinge, *Subtle Energy*, 19-20.

19. Collinge, *Subtle Energy*.

20. Ibid., 20-21.

21. Ibid., 26.

22. Ibid., 29.

23. Ibid., 30.

24. Ibid.

25. Gerber, *Vibrational Medicine*, 128.

26. Ibid., 131.

27. Ibid.

28. Ibid.

29. Ibid.

30. Ibid.

31. Ibid.

32. Ibid.

33. Judith, A. 1996. *Eastern Body, Western Mind: Psychology and the Chakra System as a Path to the Self.* Berkeley, CA: Ten Speed Press.

34. Ibid., 52.

35. Ibid.

36. Ibid., 53.

37. Ibid.

38. Myss, *Anatomy of the Spirit*, 97.

39. Flora, M. 1993. *Chakras: Key to Spiritual Opening.* Everett, WA: CDM Publications. 24.

40. Judith, *Eastern Body, Western Mind*, 106.

41. Myss, *Anatomy of the Spirit*, 97.

42. Roth, G. **http://www.gabrielleroth.com/**.

43. Judith, *Eastern Body, Western Mind*, 170.

44. Ibid., 171.

45. Myss, *Anatomy of the Spirit*, 97.

46. Myss, C. 2001. *Energy Anatomy: The Science of Power, Spirituality, and Health.* [Compact disc]. Sounds True Publishers.

47. Myss, *Anatomy of the Spirit*.

48. Ibid.

49. Judith, *Eastern Body, Western Mind*, 229.

50. Ibid.

51. Myss, *Anatomy of the Spirit*, 99.

52. Ibid.

53. Pearsall, P. 1998. *The Heart's Code: Tapping the Wisdom and Power of Our Heart Energy*. New York: Broadway Books.

54. Radha, *Realities of the Dreaming Mind*.

55. Judith, *Eastern Body, Western Mind*, 298.

56. Myss, *Anatomy of the Spirit*, 99.

57. Halpern, S. 2007. *Initiation: Inside the Great Pyramid*. [Compact disc]. Steven Halpern's Inner Peace Music.

58. Judith, *Eastern Body, Western Mind*, 352.

59. Myss, *Anatomy of the Spirit*, 99.

60. Radha, *Realities of the Dreaming Mind*.

61. Virtue, D. 2008. Angel Therapy Practitioner® workshop. Kailua-Kona, Hawaii, November 6-10. Angel Therapy, Inc. **http://www.angeltherapy.com/**.

62. Judith, *Eastern Body, Western Mind*, 406.

63. Prechtel, M. 1998. *Secrets of the Talking Jaguar: A Mayan Shaman's Journey to the Heart of the Indigenous Soul*. New York: Tarcher/Putnam.

Week Eleven: Energy Medicine

1. Hawkins, D.R. 2003. *Power vs. Force: The Hidden Determinants of Human Behavior*. Carlsbad, CA: Hay House.

2. Dyer, W. 2001. *There is a Spiritual Solution to Every Problem*. [Compact disc]. Carlsbad, CA: Hay House.

3. Hawkins, *Power vs. Force*, 2.

4. Ibid., 3.

5. Ibid.

6. Ibid., 5

7. Eden, D. 1999. *Energy Medicine*. USA: Penguin.

8. Ibid., 69.

9. Ibid.

10. Ibid., 70.

11. Hawkins, *Power vs. Force*, 30.

12. Ibid.

13. Ibid.

14. Ibid., 55.

15. Ibid.

16. Ibid.

17. Ibid., 56.

18. Ibid., 68-69

19. Ibid., 61.

20. Ibid.

21. Ibid.

22. Ibid.

23. Swanson, R. roswan@me.com. 1704 W North Five Mile Rd. Spokane WA. 99208-7112.

24. Eden, *Energy Medicine*.

25. Ibid., 98.

26. US National Institute of Health. "Acupuncture." **http://nccam.nih.gov/ health/acupuncture/acupuncture-for-pain.htm**.

27. Gerber, *Vibrational Medicine*, 241.

28. Ibid.

29. Ibid., 243.

30. Ibid.

31. Ibid., 244.

32. Ibid.

33. Ibid.

34. Ibid.

35. Ibid.

36. Ibid., 245.

37. Ibid., 246.

38. Ibid.

39. Ibid.

40. Ibid.

41. Ibid. 248.

42. Ibid. 264.

43. Gurudas. 1986. *Flower Essences and Vibrational Healing*. San Rafael, CA: Cassandra Press.

44. Gerber, *Vibrational Medicine*, 264.

45. Ibid., 249.

46. Ibid., 264.

47. Kaminski, P. n.d. "Choosing Flower Essence: An Assessment Guide." **htttp://www.fesflowers.com/choosing.htm**.

48. The Bach Centre. "Vervain." **http://www.bachcentre.com/centre/38/ vervain.htm**.

49. Smith, L. 2007. *Sent to Heal and Anoint: The Use of Essential Oils with Healing Touch Spiritual Ministry: Student notebook*. Arvada, CO: HTSM Press. 13.

50. Ibid.

51. Friedman, T. S. 1998. *Freedom through Health.* Northglen, CO: Harvest Publishing. 62.

52. Ibid.

53. Smith, *Sent to Heal and Anoint*, 18.

54. Ibid., 18.

55. Ibid.

56. Young Living Essential Oils. "Grounding." **http://cc.younglivingworld.com/ products/.**

57. Battaglia, S. 2003. *The Complete Guide to Aromatherapy.* 2nd ed. Brisbane, Australia: The International Centre of Holistic Aromatherapy. 135-137.

58. Young Living Essential Oils. "Peppermint." **http://cc.younglivingworld.com/ products/.**

59. Battaglia, *The Complete Guide to Aromatherapy*, 136.

60. Young Living Essential Oils. "Rosemary and Peppermint." **http://cc.young livingworld.com/MainFrame.asp?BodyFrame=resources/Oi lStory_main.asp**.

61. Battaglia, *The Complete Guide to Aromatherapy*, 136.

62. Ibid., 137.

63. Quigley, A. & Quigley C. 2008. *Quick Reference Guide for Using Essential Oils.* Spanish Fork, UT: Abundant Health.

64. Gerber, *Vibrational Medicine*, 338.

65. Ibid., 338-339.

66. Ibid., 564.

67. Lightwalker, C. 2003. Crystal and Stone Home Study Course. **http://the familyoflight.com**.

68. Gerber, *Vibrational Medicine*, 349.

69. Ibid., 353.

70. Ibid., 354.

71. Ibid., 355.

72. Ibid., 354.

73. Ibid., 355.

74. Ibid.

75. Ibid.

76. Ibid., 357-358.

77. Eden, *Energy Medicine*, 82-83.

78. Ibid., 82.

79. Ibid., 64.

80. Ibid., 82.

81. Ibid., 282.

82. Gach, M., & Marco, C. 1981. *Acu-Yoga: Self-Help Techniques to Relieve Tension*. Tokyo: Japan Publications (U.S.A.), Inc.

Week Twelve: Integrate and Receive

1. Mentgen, J. Healing Touch. **http://www.healingtouchprogram.com/**.

About the Author

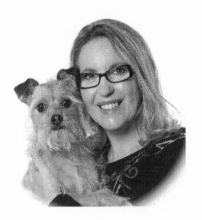

Candess M. Campbell, PhD is an international spiritual teacher, intuitive soul coach, consultant and reader, workshop facilitator, hypnotherapist, Reiki Master, and energy healer. She is also a licensed mental health counselor and chemical dependency professional with a private practice in Spokane, Washington. She specializes in assisting others to activate their energy field, their personal relationships, and their business to re-gain their own personal power and live a life of abundance, happiness, and joy.

At the core of her business, Vesta Enterprises, Incorporated, is the belief that all healing is self-healing and that becoming conscious and making positive changes increases one's personal power and enjoyment of life. She also believes that people grow and benefit from feeling safe and allowing themselves to receive. Her lifelong work has been to bridge spirituality and mainstream beliefs.

She has a large following in the US, Japan, Sweden and other countries. She has a PhD in Clinical Hypnotherapy from APU and a Masters in Counseling Psychology from Gonzaga University.

Made in the USA
Lexington, KY
06 November 2013